The Digest Book Of
PHYSICAL FITNESS

By
George B. Anderson
and
Pamela J. Johnson

DBI BOOKS, INC./NORTHFIELD, ILLINOIS

**The Digest Book of
Physical Fitness
Editorial Staff**

EDITORIAL CONSULTANT
Ron Wellman,
Director of Athletics,
Elmhurst College

PHOTOGRAPHY
John Hanusin,
Reams-Hanusin Studios

MODELS
Linda Turney
William J. Factor

ASSOCIATE PUBLISHER
Sheldon L. Factor

Table of Contents

Introduction **4**

Chapter 1: **How Physically Fit Are You?** **5**
    Personal Fitness Evaluation **6**
    The Three Basic Body Types **11**
    Methods of Exercise **12**

Chapter 2: **Developing Flexibility** **14**
    The Importance of Flexibility Fitness **14**
    Exercises for Warm-Up and
       Cooling-Off **15**
    A Program of Flexibility Exercises . . **16**

Chapter 3: **Muscular Strength** **28**
    Strength Developing Exercises
       Isometrics **30**
       Isotonics (Calisthenics) **37**
       Isotonics (Weight Training) . **41**
       Isokinetics **49**

Chapter 4: **Endurance (Muscular, Heart-Lung)** **56**
    Skeletal Muscle Endurance **56**
    Cardiovascular Endurance **57**
    Running and Jogging **60**
    Bicycling **68**
    Swimming **69**
    Rope Jumping **73**

Chapter 5: **Total Fitness Programs** **74**
    Adult Physical Fitness Programs **74**
       An Orientation Program **76**
       The Five Fitness Levels
         Program **79**
       Alternative Water Activities . **91**
       Adult Walk-Jog-Run
         Programs **93**

Introduction

EVERYONE AGREES that physical fitness is a good thing. Argue *against* it and you'll be a minority of one.

Nearly everyone also agrees that most of us don't get enough regular, healthful exercise. This same majority believes exercise is "good for you" and that they should get into better physical shape and then follow a regimen that will keep them physically fit.

So what? The same people unanimously agree that taxes are too high, that the price of gas is exorbitant, that the weather leaves a lot to be desired, and that there's too much red tape in government. Having agreed on all of these problems, having acknowledged that they exist, most of us do absolutely nothing to remedy the situation.

Yes, there are many perplexing problems—but the problem of physical fitness is a comparatively easy one to solve. However, to do it, every individual must take that first step—from awareness to action. Regular exercise is something that most of us agree we *should* do—and even *will* do—but not today, maybe tomorrow, or next week, or next month, or next year.

Getting started is the important thing, and getting started requires that you first indoctrinate yourself with a health philosophy. First, you accept the fact that you need more exercise—a fact you quickly admit and can hardly avoid. But getting started is work—and *not* working is easier than working. It isn't as pleasant as loafing. For that reason, many of us have an anti-exercise prejudice. To overcome that prejudice, all we have to do is ask ourselves four questions.

1. Would I rather be a physical mess than a healthy person?

2. Would I rather look trim and presentable or sloppy and run-down?

3. Do I want to take the high risk gamble of cardiovascular disease, high blood pressure and hypertension that menace people who don't get sufficient exercise?

4. Do I want to be physically old at an early age?

Experience has shown me that most people can read those four questions and not be bothered at all. It isn't *enough* just to read them. Right now, go back and ask yourself every one of the four questions and give your answer *out loud*.

Of course, you don't always *know* when you need more exercise. Just yesterday, I learned that a successful stockbroker I greatly admire is in the cardiac care unit of a nearby hospital, after having suffered a serious heart attack that came without warning.

It was a shock, because this man had always *looked* healthy. He burned up a lot of energy on the job. But after he gets out of the hospital, which I certainly hope he does, he'll be faced with the vital necessity of a cardiovascular-pulmonary rebuilding program that will call for regular, vigorous exercise. Because he's a smart man, he'll follow the doctor's advice. And that brings up an important thing about your physical fitness starting program. It must be one you can live with comfortably—one that's not downright unpleasant for you. For most of us, the *only* way we'll embrace a fitness program we don't like is to be scared into it.

However, before you begin a physical fitness program you should take that first step which is a *must* for most of us—a physical examination.

George B. Anderson

CHAPTER 1

How Physically Fit Are You?

THE FIRST STEP, an absolute must, is a consultation with your family doctor or a visit to a physical fitness evaluation center. If you're as lax about regular physical examinations as most people are, a complete physical would be in order. Most of us are unaware of our true physical conditions and therefore run the risk of injuring ourselves by embarking on an exercise program which may be too strenuous. If you are *under 30,* have had a physical exam in the past year and the doctor found nothing wrong with you, you can start exercising. If you are *30-59,* you should have a medical checkup at least 3-4 months prior to beginning an exercise program. In all cases, an EKG should be taken while you're exercising. *Over 59* have a checkup, including an EKG, immediately prior to embarking on an exercise program. In addition, for those who are overweight, have a history of high blood pressure or heart trouble, an exercise program should *never* be begun without your doctor's approval.

The physical exam should include examination of your blood pressure, cardiovascular system, condition of your muscles and joints and a blood test for cholesterol and triglycerides.

The doctor is all in favor of your starting and keeping with a physical fitness program. He's also in a position to know if any of the forms of exercise you have in mind would be unwise for you. You should also ask him if there's any particular kind of exercise he thinks you need to stress. Find out your major physical weaknesses and ask him if he'd suggest corrective exercises to alleviate them.

Unfortunately, some doctors are overworked and are much too busy to spend any length of time with their patients unless they feel it's absolutely necessary. For that reason, it's a good idea to have a written list of questions for the doctor to answer. By having such a list, you'll be able to confine your visit to the physician to the items which concern you.

You'll probably have specific questions in addition to these, but here's a basic list for a starter:

1. Do I have any physical condition for which any type of exercise could be dangerous? What is it? Do you know of any corrective exercises?

2. Do I need to lose any weight? How much? What kind of diet would you recommend to accomplish such a weight loss?

3. How are my heart and pulse? What's my blood pressure? What effect should these things have on an exercise program?

4. Is my back all right? How about my kidneys?

5. Do I have to worry about my legs, kneecaps or hip joints? What kind of exercise would be harmful for them?

6. Do I have any indication of diabetes? What effect should it have on my exercise program?

The medical doctor can definitely establish the state of your physical health. Then, to give you good advice, he must know the type of physical fitness program you want to start with, and whether it will have a light or strenuous start.

He can come close to estimating the physical tolerance of your body, but once he has done that, you, yourself, can be the best judge of when you're approaching the limit of your physical tolerance. That tolerance, of course, depends on your age as well as your physical condition.

The Stress Test

As mentioned above, your physical checkup should include an EKG while you are engaged in a physical activity. (An EKG taken while at rest really does not tell you how much stress your circulo-respiratory system can handle.) Why is such a test important? A stress test evaluates and tests the fitness of your heart, lungs and circulatory endurance. How long can you walk at a steady pace before your breathing becomes strained? How does your heart react to this same exercise? Is the stress too much for your heart? How efficiently is your cardiovascular-pulmonary system working? If you wish to embark on a strenuous fitness program, the answers to these questions could be *very* important.

Usually the stress test takes one of two forms—the individual pedals a stationary bicycle or walks and/or alternately runs on a motorized treadmill while being monitored by an EKG. By watching the EKG readings, blood pressure rate and respiration rate, the doctor can tell you the limits of your physical capacity and many times prescribe a program for you to increase your cardiovascular-pulmonary endurance.

There are two major drawbacks to the stress test—lack of doctors and centers which perform these tests and the cost which can run from $100 for the stress test to $250 for a complete fitness evaluation including strength, stamina and body composition. If you can afford such a fitness analysis, first try your local hospital and see if they have a cardiologist on staff who will conduct the test. If you live in a big city, try your local YMCA or YWCA. If you live in a university town, phone their medical school or physical education department and inquire about the stress test. In addition to these sources, there are four stress test centers in the United States:

Vital Fitness Evaluation Center
1 Embarcadero Plaza
San Francisco, Calif. 94111
(415) 433-7286

Institute for Aerobics Research
12100 Preston Road
Dallas, Tex. 75230
(214) 239-7223

George Sheehan
Stress Testing Program
Riverview Hospital
Red Bank, N.J. 07701
(201) 741-2700

Cardio-Metrics Institute
295 Madison Avenue
New York, NY 10017
(212) 889-6123

PERSONAL FITNESS EVALUATION

Most of us can't afford to shell out $100 for a stress test and if that were the criterion for starting a fitness program, most of us would not think twice about starting. Fortunately, there are much simpler ways to test your cardiovascular endurance, body composition (percentage of fat), and your strength, stamina and flexibility. However, you should have your doctor's okay before trying these tests.

The Step Test

The Step Test is one of a number of tests designed to measure your cardiovascular endur-

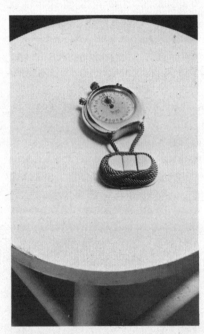

Step Test Equipment —Stopwatch and Stool

Pulse rate is taken three times

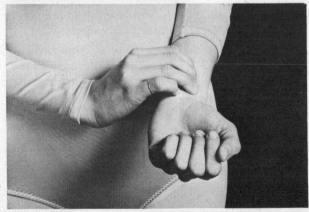

ance. By putting you through 4 minutes of strenuous exercise it will tell you how hard your heart has to work, in order to move blood through your system during the exercise and how fast it recovers from that strain. *Do not smoke or engage in any physical activity 2 hours prior to taking this test.* You will need: a bench (see chart below for correct size), and a stopwatch, wristwatch or clock with a second hand.

If You Are	The Bench Should Be
Under 5' tall	12" high
5'1" to 5'3" tall	14" high
5'3" to 5'9" tall	16" high
5'9" to 6' tall	18" high
Over 6' tall	20" high

The bench can be a chair, two stair steps, an ottoman, etc. The test consists of stepping up and down from bench to floor 30 times a minute for 4 minutes. To begin, stand facing the bench and, starting with either foot, place your foot on the bench and then step up so both feet are on the bench. Then immediately step down so both feet are on the floor. This test should be performed rhythmically so that every 2 seconds you complete the up and down motion. After 4 minutes of continuous exercise, sit down and remain quiet for 1 minute, then take your pulse rates and record them as follows:

1. Pulse rate after 1 minute after exercise, taken for 30-second period.
2. Pulse rate after 2 minutes after exercise, taken for 30-second period.
3. Pulse rate after 3 minutes after exercise, taken for 30-second period.

To determine your cardiovascular fitness, add the three pulse counts and refer to the table below.

When the three 30-second pulse counts total:	The Recovery Index is:	Then the response to this test is:
199 or more	60 or less	Poor
from 171-198	between 61-70	Average
from 150-170	between 71-80	Good
from 133-149	between 81-90	Very Good
132 or less	91 or more	Excellent

You may find that you can not complete this test. Don't get discouraged. Just rate your fitness "poor" and make up your mind to do something about it. However, if you could not complete the test and/or after the test any of these symptoms appear, it's advisable to see your doctor: excessive breathlessness long after exercise; bluing of the lips; pale or clammy skin or cold sweating; unusual fatigue; persistent shakiness or weakness 10 minutes after the exercise; muscle twitching following exercise.

Remember to record your rating for this test on the Physical Fitness Evaluation Chart (page 11). Retake this test after 2 weeks on a fitness program to see how much you have improved.

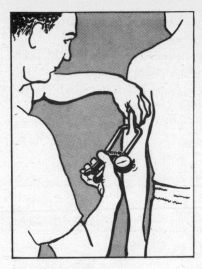

The Pinch Test

Body Fat Measurement

Body Fat Measurement will tell you if you are carrying around too much body fat; in other words, it tells you if you are obese. Although obesity is usually evident from appearances alone, appearances may be deceiving. Most of us refer to the Department of Agriculture height/build/weight chart to determine whether we are overweight or whether we fall into the normal weight range. What that chart does not tell you is how much of your weight is body fat. In the average healthy man, the total body weight is 15 percent fat, 23 percent water, 58 percent muscle and organs and 4 percent bone mineral. The percentage of body fat for a woman will be slightly higher. In the obese person, the percentage of body fat far exceeds these average amounts, so that even though your total body weight may fall in the normal range for your height and build, your percentage of body fat may be too high.

Most of us are aware of the dangers we face if there is excess fat in the body—increased chance of heart disease, high blood pressure, diabetes, etc. How can you tell whether you are carrying around too much body fat?

Pinch Test: This test can be done by your doctor who will use a measuring device called a caliper to measure the thickness of a fold of skin on the back of your arm. However, you can get a rough idea at home by gently gripping with thumb and forefinger the skin behind your upper arm midway between elbow and shoulder. If the thickness is from ¼ to ½-inch, rate yourself excellent (¼-inch) or good (½-inch). If the thickness is more than that, you have some work to do and rate yourself poor.

Weight Gain Test: Can you remember how much you weighed at the age of 25? How about at age 16? If you can, take the lower of the two weights. Your weight now if you are a light-boned person should only be 5-10 percent more and if you are a muscular or heavyset person, your weight should be 5-10 percent less. Rate yourself excellent if you passed this test and poor if you did not.

Flexibility Test

The Flexibility Test will tell you the range of motion, or lack thereof, through which your limbs are able to move. Since there are many joints in our bodies, there is no one general test which will tell you your overall flexibility fitness. However, most of us tend to lose flexibility in the hamstring, low back and neck areas first. So these are the joints to be tested with the Sitting Stretch Test.

Sitting Stretch: Put two pieces of tape on the floor about 5 inches apart and align them horizontally. Next, sit down on the floor, legs stretched out straight, toes pointing upward. Place your heels on each piece of tape. You should have a marker of some sort—a checker, backgammon chip, etc. Now bend forward, slowly stretching as far as possible. Touch the finger tips to the floor, placing the outer edge of the marker at the forward tip of the fingers. Now measure the distance between the tape and the outer edge of your marker. If you could reach 8 inches (men) or 12 inches (women) beyond the tape, your flexibility is excellent. From 5-6 inches (men) or 6-8 inches (women) is good. From 1-4 inches (men) or 1-5 inches (women) is average flexibility. Below that you need work—rate yourself poor.

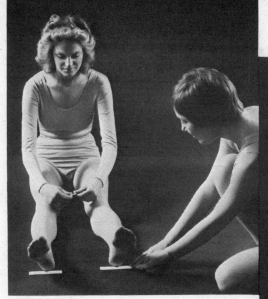
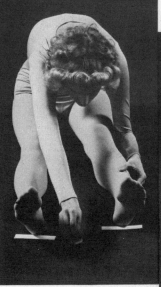
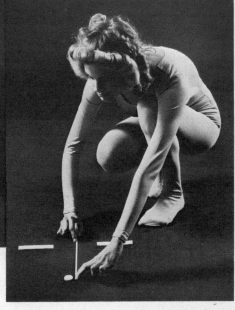

Muscular Strength Test

Muscular Strength Test does as its name implies—it tests the strength of your muscles. As was true for the Flexibility Test, there is no one general test that can determine your overall muscular strength fitness. We will test the muscles, that, as we grow older, tend to lose strength first—the abdominal muscles, shoulder and arm muscles and upper and lower back muscles. You should be able to do all three of these tests. These are the very minimum tests for strength fitness.

The failure to do even one test is an indication of very poor muscular strength. Score yourself for all three with either pass or fail.

Pushup (arm and shoulder strength): Lie face down on the floor, legs together, hands on floor palms down under shoulders with fingers pointing straight ahead. Extend arms, pushing body off the floor so that your weight rests on your hands and toes. Keeping your back straight lower your body until chest touches the floor.

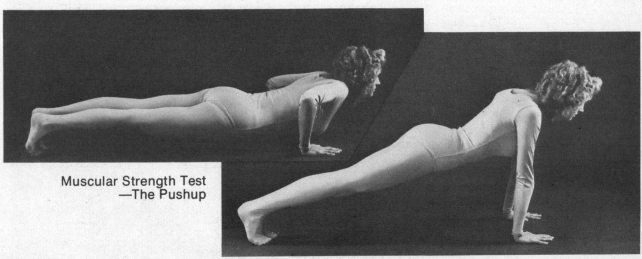

Muscular Strength Test
—The Pushup

Prone Arch (upper and lower back muscles): Lie face down, hands tucked under thighs. Arch back, raising legs and chest off the floor. Hold that position for a count of 10. *Caution:* If you have lower back problems, you should not try this test.

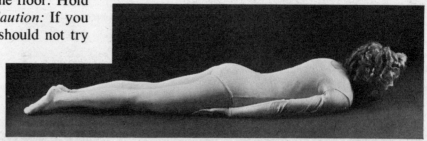

Muscular Strength Test
—The Prone Arch

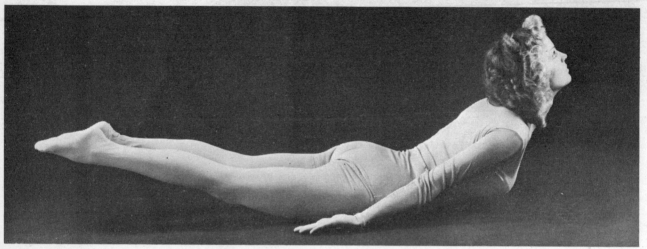

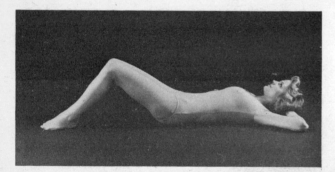

Muscular Strength Test
—The Situp

Situp (abdominal muscles): Lie on your back, legs slightly bent, feet about 1 inch apart. Tuck your toes under a sofa or have a partner hold your ankles—your heels should be in contact with the floor during the situp motion. Lace your fingers behind your neck. Curl up into the sitting position.

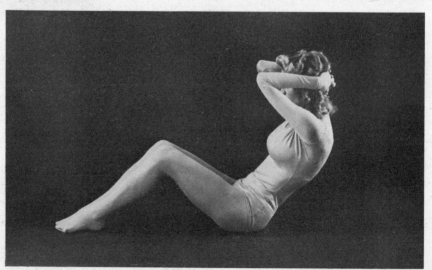

Muscular Endurance Test

Muscular Endurance Test tests the ability of a muscle to perform a specific task for a length of time. Once again, there is no one test to determine the endurance of each of your muscles. The situp, however, is the most widely accepted and used test for muscular endurance.

Situp (abdominal muscle endurance): Perform the situp as described in the Muscular Strength Test. Do as many situps as you can.

For both men and women, a score of 50 or more situps is excellent. A score of 40-49 (men), 35-49 (women) is good and a score of 25-39 (men), 22-34 (women) is average. If you could not complete 25 (men) or 22 (women) situps, you scored below average. Rate yourself poor.

PERSONAL PHYSICAL FITNESS EVALUATION CHART

How physically fit are you? This chart will help you take an overall view of your present state of physical fitness. For each of the tests you just completed, put a check mark down by your rating. You can now easily see in which areas you need the most work.

TEST	RATING
Cardiovascular Endurance	
Step Test	___ Excellent
	___ Very Good
	___ Good
	___ Average
	___ Poor
Body Fat Measurement	
Pinch Test	___ Excellent
	___ Good
	___ Poor
Weight Gain Test	___ Excellent
	___ Poor
Flexibility	
Sitting Stretch	___ Excellent
	___ Good
	___ Average
	___ Poor
Muscular Strength	
Pushup	___ Pass ___ Fail
Prone Arch	___ Pass ___ Fail
Situp	___ Pass ___ Fail
Muscular Endurance	
Situps	___ Excellent
	___ Good
	___ Average
	___ Poor

THE THREE BASIC BODY TYPES

Now that you have a pretty fair evaluation of your present physical fitness status, you have one more aspect to consider—your body type. People come in many shapes and sizes. Some are thin and wiry and others are muscular and heavy. In between is a myriad of combinations—top heavy with thin legs, bottom heavy with narrow chest and on and on. However, everyone falls into one of the three basic body types.

Why is it important to know your body type? First of all, you must face the fact that you can't do much to change your basic body type—no matter how much training or exercise you do. If you fall into the thin muscled and boned, slender body type, no amount of weight training is going to turn you into an Arnold Schwartzenegger. In fact, weight training for such a body type is usually very frustrating. There are exercises for building strength that a person with such a body type would be much more successful with. The types of exercises listed under each body type are all types of activities using large muscle groups. These are types of exercises that are best suited for that particular body type. This doesn't mean that if your body type is Endomorphic, for example, you should not or cannot jog. It simply means your body type is best suited to other types of exercises and you will be more successful in performing those than you will in attempting to jog.

Endomorph: The endomorph has noticeable soft musculature with a round face, short neck, double chin and wide hips. There is little muscle development and small bones.

Exercises: Exercises best suited to the endomorph are bowling, bicycling, swimming, tennis and badminton.

Mesomorph: The mesomorph is solid, muscular, big-boned and rugged. Generally of medium height with large chest, slender waist, long torso and short powerful legs.

Exercises: Exercises best suited to the mesomorph are bowling, bicycling, golf, handball, weight training, swimming, jogging, hiking.

Ectomorph: The ectomorph has a slender body, is thin muscled and thin boned, has a long slender neck, narrow chest and has very little body fat.

Exercises: Exercises best suited to the ectomorph are badminton, basketball, bicycling, golf, hiking, jogging, tennis and running.

METHODS OF EXERCISE

Now that you know what your present state of physical fitness is and the types of large muscled activities best suited to your body type, let's look at the methods of exercise you will be using to improve your fitness. There are five basic methods of exercise—**aerobics, calisthenics, isometrics, isotonics** and **isokinetics.** Each method has its followers and its detractors. For the purposes of this book, we recognize that each of these exercise methods helps the individual build and improve one or more aspects of the total fitness spectrum—*flexibility, muscle strength, muscle endurance* and *cardiovascular-pulmonary endurance.* However, no one method can be used as a total fitness program. No one method is best suited to improve all four aspects of the total fitness spectrum.

Aerobic Exercises

Aerobic exercise is any rhythmical activity that causes a sustained increase in heart rate, respiration and muscle metabolism. Such exercise will improve the efficiency and the capacity of the cardiovascular and respiratory system—heart, lungs, and blood vessels. Aerobic exercise is essential to any total fitness program because no other exercise method effectively builds the strength and endurance of the cardiovascular-pulmonary system. This exercise method includes such activities as jogging, swimming, bicycling, walking, running in place, jumping rope.

In order to benefit from any aerobic exercise, you must increase your heart beat rate to a training rate of 110-178 beats per minute depending on your age and fitness evaluation* (see chart below) and sustain that heart beat rate for a minimum of 15 minutes. The best way to judge if you have reached your training heart rate is to do 5 minutes of strenuous aerobic exercise and then immediately take your pulse for 15 seconds. Multiply that number by four. If your heart rate is below that suggested, you should pick up your pace—i.e., if jogging, jog at a faster pace. If your rate is higher than suggested, slow down your exercise pace. You should not over-stress your heart.

---

*Your fitness evaluation can be determined by your Step Test rating. Refer to the preceding Personal Physical Fitness Evaluation Chart.

Aerobic Fitness Training Heart Rates

Fitness Level	Training Rate (Intensity) (in beats/min)
Excellent	
Age 20	164-178
25	162-176
30	160-174
35	157-171
40	154-168
45	151-164
50	148-161
55	145-158
60	143-155
Average	
Age 20	153-164
25	151-162
30	148-159
35	145-157
40	142-154
45	139-151
50	136-149
55	133-146
60	130-143
Poor	
Age 20	140-154
25	137-151
30	134-148
35	130-144
40	126-140
45	122-136
50	118-132
55	114-128
60	110-124

When you take the count, if your heart rate is around 30 beats over the suggested training rate, you've reached your maximum heart beat rate. Slow down your exercise pace. Take another count after another 5 minutes of aerobic exercise to see if you are within your training heart beat range.

There are other exercises which will help cardiovascular-pulmonary endurance. Handball, racquetball, basketball and tennis will all produce the desired results if the exercise is steady and continuous over a period of time. The key words here are steady and continuous. If you are playing tennis and after 5 minutes take a breather you are not helping to strengthen your heart and respiratory systems. In that 5 minutes you may have increased your heart beat rate to the proper training level but, when you stop, that rate drops rapidly. It is suggested that these sports activities be used only for maintenance of aerobic fitness, not as a substitute.

Calisthenics

Most of us have done some sort of calisthenic exercise—the jumping jack, pushups, situps, etc. Calisthenics are systematic, rhythmic bodily exercises usually without apparatus. If calisthenic exercises are used to build only strength and endurance, then calishthenics is considered to be *isotonic* exercise. However, calisthenics can be considered an exercise method unto itself and as such can build cardiopulmonary endurance, increase muscle strength and endurance and increase flexibility. In other words, calisthenics, if used properly, can be implemented as a total fitness program although it is not generally recommended. To be used as a total fitness program, the exercise series you choose must be carried out in a steady and continuous fashion with no rest between exercises. If between exercises a "rest" period is needed, then only walking or running in place are acceptable.

Calisthenics in combination with other methods of exercise is the most effective way to utilize this exercise method. The reason being—using calisthenics to build muscular strength, for example, would take much longer than a weight training program. The same can be said for calisthenics and cardiovascular pulmonary endurance. The amount and vigor of calisthenics required to increase your heart beat rate to the training level and then sustain that level is much harder work than a 15-30 minute walk, jog, swim or bicycle ride. It is generally recognized that calisthenics are not as effective as aerobic exercises in building cardiovascular-pulmonary endurance.

Calisthenics can be used effectively to correct special problems or to develop selected areas of the body.

Isometrics/Isotonics/Isokinetics

Isometric exercises involve the contraction of muscles *without* movement. In isometric exercises a muscle or group of muscles is exerted against an immovable force such as a wall or another set of muscles. A good example would be putting your hands together in front of you and pushing them together as hard as possible. Isometrics are most effective in building muscle strength and tone.

Isotonic exercises involve muscle contractions *with* movement. Weight training would be a good example of isotonic exercise. Isotonics are used most effectively in building muscular strength and endurance.

Isokinetic exercises require movement with a *controlled resistance*. Usually, isokinetic exercises involve the use of exercising machines. The machine controls the amount of resistance—at a slow speed there is little resistance but as you increase in speed, the resistance is also increased. Isokinetics is the best of the three for building muscle strength.

Isometrics, isotonics and isokinetics will build muscular strength, endurance and all over body tone. However, none of these should be considered a total fitness program because they do not stimulate the cardiovascular system and therefore do not build cardiovascular-pulmonary endurance. They also do not provide any flexibility improvement. These three exercise methods, however, can be effective as an integral part of a total fitness program.

Hopefully, you're now eager to start a total fitness program—but don't be impatient. Before we give you any actual programs, we want to give you a basic knowledge of the four aspects of physical fitness—**Flexibility** *Chapter 2*, **Muscular Strength** *Chapter 3,* **Muscle Endurance** and **Cardiovascular-Pulmonary Endurance** *Chapter 4*—why you need to develop each aspect and what exercises you can do to attain fitness in each aspect.

CHAPTER 2

Developing Flexibility

AS STATED IN Chapter 1, flexibility pertains to the range of motion you have in a particular joint or series of joints. That range of motion is controlled by the degree the muscles, connective tissue, tendons, ligaments and skin associated to that particular joint can be stretched. In doing flexibility exercises the purpose is to increase the elasticity of the muscles and connective tissue surrounding a particular joint so you get the maximum range of motion.

IMPORTANCE OF FLEXIBILITY FITNESS

All-Over Fitness

Good flexibility fitness contributes to your overall fitness—your movements become more graceful and your chances of injuring yourself in everyday life are lessened. However, for many of us our inactive life-style leads to inflexibility in major joints in the body. The areas of the body which lose flexibility first are the hamstrings, lower back, neck and pectoral areas. These are the joints most susceptible to injury by being forced beyond their normal range of motion. Your "normal" range depends on your flexibility fitness. Millions of Americans are beset by lower back problems which in most cases are caused by the lack of physical activity, poor posture, inadequate flexibility and weak abdominal and/or lower back muscles. We've all encountered situations when we've had to make a sudden movement which overstressed a muscle—perhaps lifting something that was really too heavy for us—which resulted in either muscle soreness or something more serious such as a torn ligament or a sprained or torn muscle. Good flexibility

What is Flexibility?

Flexibility is but one of the four basic elements of the total physical fitness spectrum—but it is an essential element for development of strength and endurance. Inadequate flexibility when performing strength and endurance exercises can prove harmful and in some cases such exercises performed without proper warm-up can actually reduce the range of motion you have in your joints. It's not necessary that you possess above-normal flexibility—in fact, extreme flexibility coupled with inadequate muscular strength can be detrimental. But a reasonable or average range of motion in each body joint is important for everyday living and esstential for participation in a total fitness program.

fitness will neither prevent muscle soreness nor prevent a more serious muscle or tendon injury. But it will reduce your chances of such an injury by increasing the degree to which your muscles and tendons can be stretched before injury is incurred.

Graceful body movement and better posture can also be benefits of flexibility fitness. As we grow older, our muscles, ligaments and tendons begin to lose some of their elasticity and connective tissues become stiff and actually shorten. The result is a loss in the range of motion in the joints. Without adequate joint flexibility, body movements, whether walking, sitting or during sports activity, become jerky and lack smoothness of action. In addition to poor body movement our posture can suffer from a combination of muscle strength loss and inadequate flexibility. Chest and shoulder muscles which become weak rely on connective tissue to keep the shoulders from pulling forward. However, connective tissue becomes stiff and shortens, only aggravating the problem/and a round shouldered posture results.

The good news is that if you do suffer from poor posture and lack a gracefulness in movement, it is reversible. If you already possess good posture and move smoothly, *also* is reversible. Flexibility exercises are essential to improve and maintain our physical appearance.

Flexibility Exercises for Warm-Up

In any fitness program there are four periods of exercise which make up the total program—warm-up, conditioning activities, circulatory activities and cooling-off. All are vital—none should be ignored:

The warm-up period, which should last from 5-10 minutes, stretches and limbers up the muscles and speeds up the action of the heart (hopefully to training rate) and lungs. It prepares the body for greater exertion and reduces the possibility of unnecessary strain.

The conditioning period builds and increases flexibility, muscle strength and endurance and tones up abdominal, back, leg, arm and other major muscles.

The circulatory activity period produces contractions of large muscle groups for relatively longer periods than the conditioning activities—to stimulate and strengthen the circulatory and respiratory systems.

The cooling-off period is essential in helping the body—in particular, the muscles, heart and lungs—return to its normal activity level.

The most effective way of using flexibility exercises is to include them in the warm-up and cooling-off periods. Flexibility exercises used in warm-up activities prepare you for the vigorous conditioning period by stimulating blood circulation, increasing your heart rate and raising your body temperature. But most importantly, flexibility exercises stretch and limber up your muscles and joints so they can adapt to the increase in activity. The warming up of your muscles and joints increases your range of motion. If you ignore the warm-up and go head-long into vigorous exercise (e.g., jogging or weight lifting or snow shoveling) you'll be much sorer the next day than you would have been had you done

warm-up exercises—and that's if you are in decent physical condition. If you are in poor physical condition and you ignore a warm-up period before those same vigorous exercises, you could come away with something more serious than muscle soreness. Sudden vigorous stretching of a muscle causes the muscle to protect itself by a reflexive contraction or tightening up. Restretching that same muscle in a burst of activity can overstretch the muscle and result in a muscle tear or worse. Most of us have experienced to a much lesser degree the unpleasant effects of this reflexive contraction when, after a long period of inactivity, we decide to go out for a long run. The next day finds us virtual cripples. How much wiser to have spent a few days doing flexibility exercises and then preceded the run with a warm-up exercise period.

When selecting flexibility exercises for your warm-up period, keep in mind that flexibility is specific to each joint. Each joint should be exercised with particular attention to those joints you know will receive the most strain when you begin your conditioning period of exercise.

Cooling-Off Exercises

Flexibility exercises used in the cooling-off period following vigorous exercise do the reverse of the warm-up exercises. Instead of preparing your body for vigorous activity, they help your body return gradually to its normal working level. Failing to do cooling-off exercises can result in lightheadedness, dizziness and sometimes even nausea. The reason for this is simple. While engaged in vigorous activity your heart beats rapidly, supplying the extra oxygen the muscles need for the stepped-up acitivity. When you suddenly stop exercising with no cooling-off period, your heart rate drops rapidly but is still beating far above its normal level. The additional blood is still being pumped to the now inactive muscles. This leaves less blood to supply the brain with oxygen—therefore the lightheaded or dizzy feeling. A cooling-off period following vigorous exercise allows your heart to slow down gradually and your circulatory system to adapt to the lesser demands of normal activity.

If you want the greatest possible benefit from flexibility exercises, the cooling-off period is ideal. Your muscles, tendons and ligaments are warmed up and stimulated by the conditioning and circulatory periods. In this condition your muscles are more pliable and can most easily be stretched. By doing flexibility exercises in the cooling-off period you can work on stretching your muscles so that a reflexive muscle contraction is prevented. This post-conditioning stretching not only speeds you to flexibility fitness but will help reduce muscle soreness and cramps.

FLEXIBILITY EXERCISES

In doing the following flexibility exercises, it is important you remember to move slowly. You want to stretch your muscles, not pull or tear them. For example, when doing the Seated Toe Touches, lean *slowly* forward, trying to touch your fingers to your toes and then gently pull forward further to stretch the muscles. A jerking or vigorous bobbing will only tighten the muscles through the muscle's protective reflex contraction. If, when you begin, you're not sure if you are doing the exercises too vigorously—wait 24 hours. You'll get your answer.

The exercise method which best helps build flexibility fitness is calisthenics. Among the calisthenic exercises there will be considerable overlapping with exercises that help the flexibility fitness of the same muscle or groups of muscles. After the name of each exercise is the muscle or groups of muscles that the exercise helps. This allows you a choice of exercises—after all, we all have our personal preferences.

Calisthenic Exercises

HAMSTRING STRETCH (lower back and hamstring muscles, hip joints)

1. Stand erect. Cross your right leg over the straight left leg and plant your right foot firmly on the floor.
2. Put your right palm firmly on your left shoulder with the right elbow projecting downward toward your navel. Your left arm should be hanging at your side.
3. Keeping your left leg straight, bend slowly forward, bringing your right elbow as close to your crossed legs as you can get it. The straight left arm arcs backward as you do this. Tighten your abdominal muscles as you bend forward.
4. Return to starting position.
5. Repeat the exercise to the opposite side, with left palm on right shoulder and left leg crossed over the right.

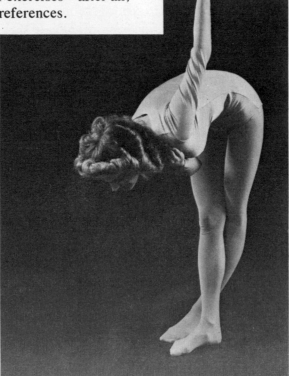
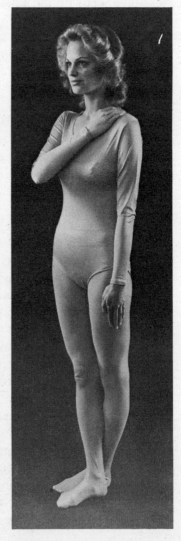

The Hamstring Stretch

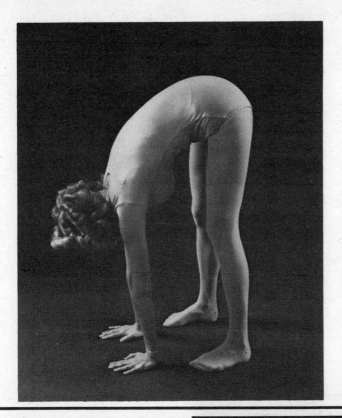

FLEXED LEG BACK STRETCH (thigh, hamstring and lower back muscles)

1. Stand with knees slightly flexed, feet shoulder width apart, hands at sides.
2. Slowly bend over, touching the floor with the palms of your hands.
3. Now slowly try to straighten your legs without lifting your palms off the floor.
4. Return to starting position.

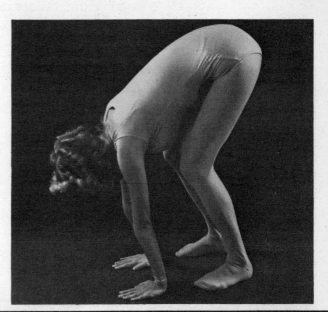

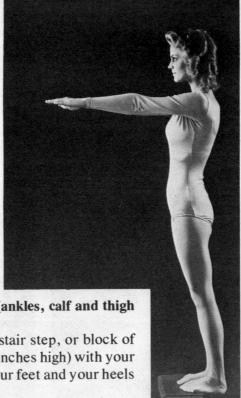

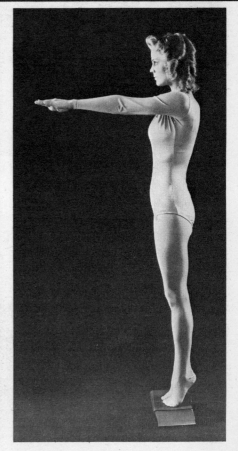

LOWER LEG STRETCH (ankles, calf and thigh muscles)

1. Stand on a thick book, stair step, or block of wood (approximately 6 inches high) with your weight on the balls of your feet and your heels raised.
2. Lower heels trying to touch the floor.
3. Return to starting position.

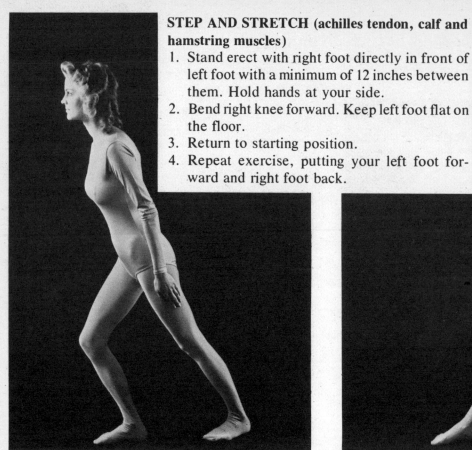
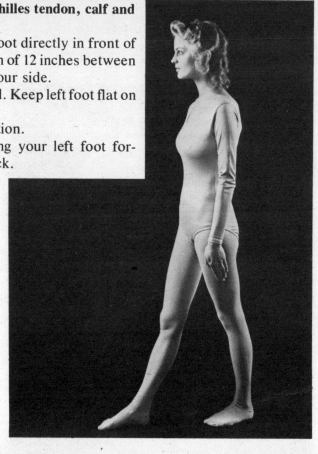

STEP AND STRETCH (achilles tendon, calf and hamstring muscles)

1. Stand erect with right foot directly in front of left foot with a minimum of 12 inches between them. Hold hands at your side.
2. Bend right knee forward. Keep left foot flat on the floor.
3. Return to starting position.
4. Repeat exercise, putting your left foot forward and right foot back.

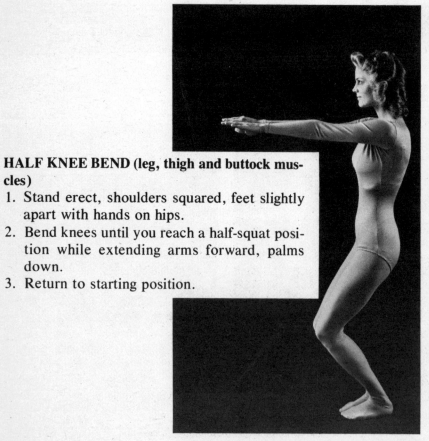
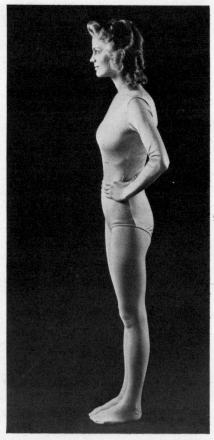

HALF KNEE BEND (leg, thigh and buttock muscles)

1. Stand erect, shoulders squared, feet slightly apart with hands on hips.
2. Bend knees until you reach a half-squat position while extending arms forward, palms down.
3. Return to starting position.

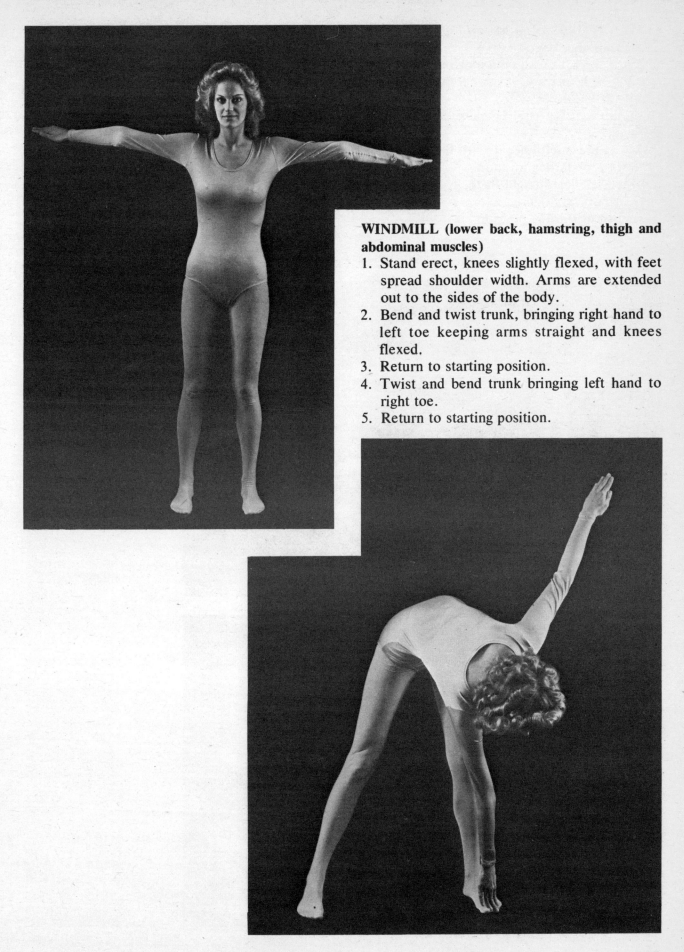

WINDMILL (lower back, hamstring, thigh and abdominal muscles)

1. Stand erect, knees slightly flexed, with feet spread shoulder width. Arms are extended out to the sides of the body.
2. Bend and twist trunk, bringing right hand to left toe keeping arms straight and knees flexed.
3. Return to starting position.
4. Twist and bend trunk bringing left hand to right toe.
5. Return to starting position.

STRIDE STRETCH (wrist, hip, groin, leg and lower back muscles)

1. Squat on floor with buttocks touching heels, body bent forward, hands on floor on either side of knees.
2. Move right leg straight back, keeping back rigid.
3. Try to press left knee toward the floor.
4. Return to starting position.
5. Move left leg straight back, trying to press right knee to floor.
6. Return to starting position.

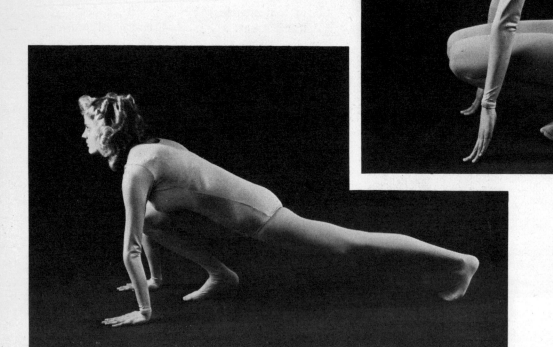

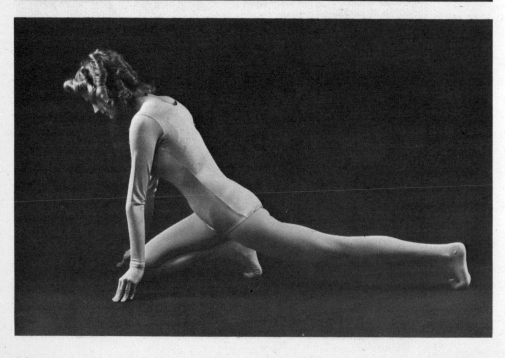

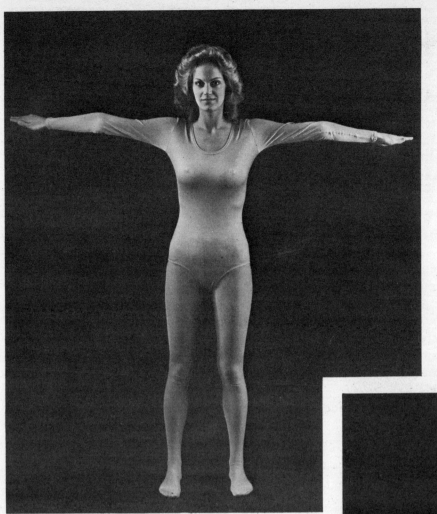

SIDE TWISTER (trunk, shoulder and back muscles)

1. Stand erect, feet about 12 inches apart, arms extended out to the sides with palms down.
2. Twist torso as far as possible to the left keeping arms extended.
3. Repeat, turning torso as far as possible to the right, keeping arms extended.
4. Return to starting position.

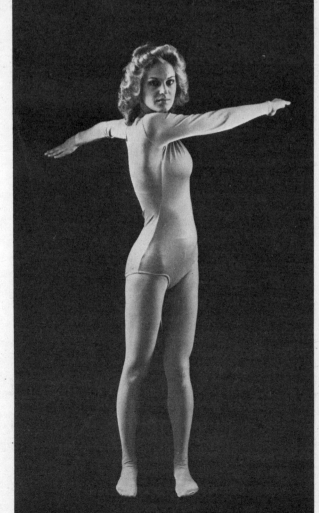

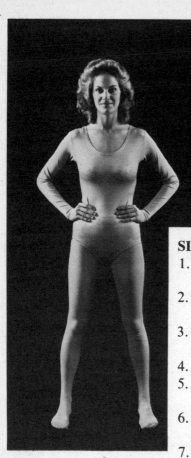

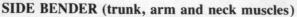

SIDE BENDER (trunk, arm and neck muscles)

1. Stand erect with hands on hips and feet about shoulder width apart.
2. Extend left arm overhead, keeping right hand on hip.
3. Bend to the right side as far as possible and gently pull.
4. Return to starting position.
5. Extend right arm overhead, keeping left hand on hip.
6. Bend to the left side as far as possible and gently pull.
7. Return to starting position.

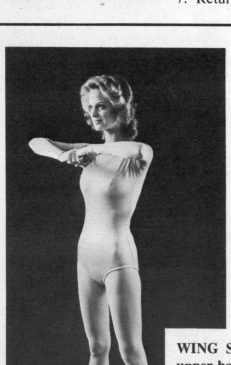

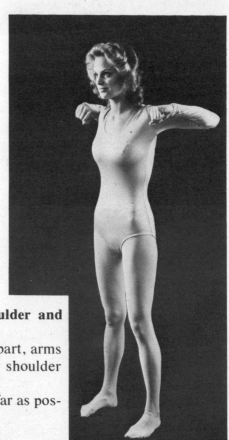

WING STRETCHER (pectoral, shoulder and upper back muscles)

1. Stand erect, feet about 12 inches apart, arms bent, elbows out to each side at shoulder height.
2. Slowly push elbows backwards as far as possible.
3. Return to starting position.

NECK CIRCLES (neck muscles)

1. Stand erect with arms hanging loosely at sides.
2. Bend neck forward until chin touches chest.
3. Turn head to the right as far as possible.
4. Bend neck backward as far as possible.
5. Turn head to the left as far as possible.
6. Gently roll head in full circle, first to the right and then again to the left.

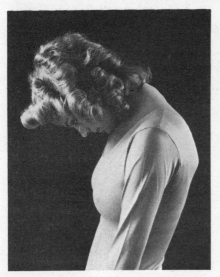
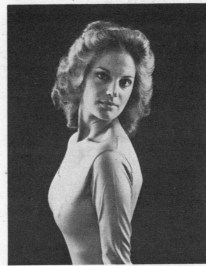
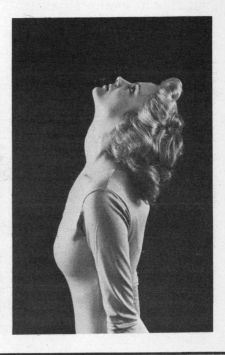

HURDLE STRETCH (lower leg, thigh, abdominal and back muscles)

1. Sit on floor with left leg extended out front and right leg bent at knee and out to the side. Hands should be at your sides.
2. Reach out with right hand and touch extended left toe.
3. Return to starting position.
4. Reverse position of legs with right leg extended and left leg bent at the knee and out the side.
5. Reach out with left hand and touch extended right toe.
6. Return to starting position.

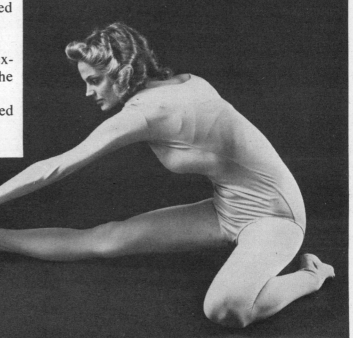

SIT AND STRETCH (lower back, inner thigh and hamstring muscles)

1. Sit on floor, legs spread with knees straight. Clasp hands behind neck.
2. Bend forward at waist as far as possible.
3. Gently stretch, trying to touch elbows to floor.
4. Return to starting position.

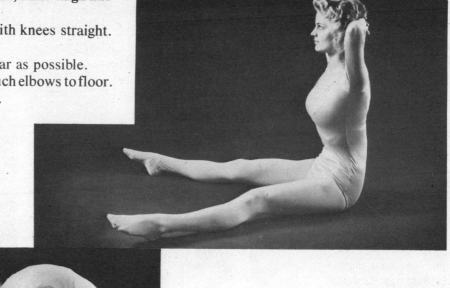

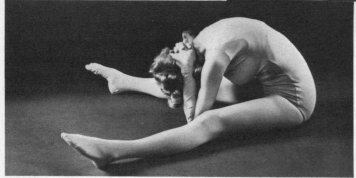

SIDE LUNGE (inside and outside thigh muscles)

1. In a squat position, move your right leg out to the side.
2. Keeping your right leg straight, gently push right leg out as far as possible.
3. Return to squat position.
4. Extend left leg out to the side.
5. Return to squat position.

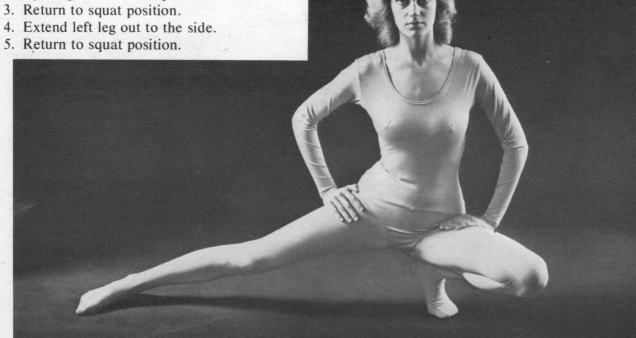

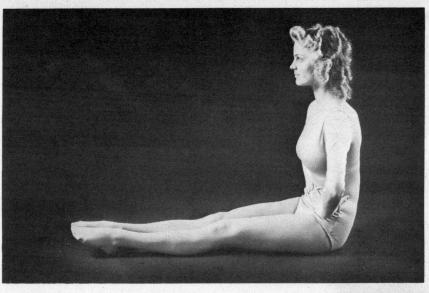

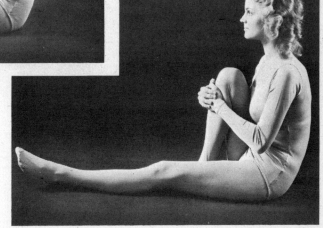

KNEE PULL (thigh and trunk muscles)

1. Sit on floor, back straight, both legs extended straight ahead.
2. Keeping back straight, pull right leg as close to chest as possible.
3. Return to starting position.
4. Pull left leg as close to chest as possible.
5. Return to starting position.

TOE PULL (groin and thigh muscles)

1. Sit on floor, knees bent and out to each side with the bottoms of your feet together and drawn as close up to your body as possible.
2. Grasp feet with both hands and pull on toes while pressing knees toward the floor with your elbows.

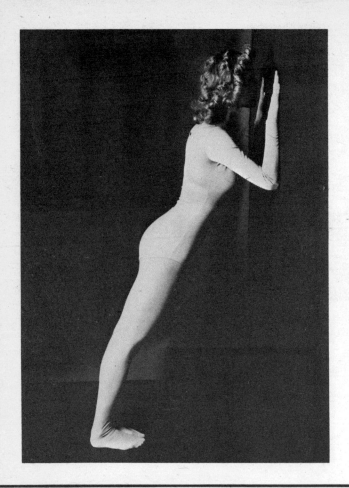

WALL STRETCH (calf and hamstring muscles)
1. Stand erect, 3 feet from a wall with feet slightly apart.
2. Put both hands on wall.
3. Keeping heels on the floor, lean forward, slowly trying to touch head to wall.
4. Return to starting position.

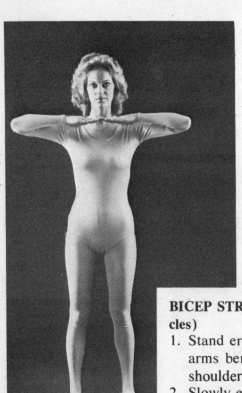

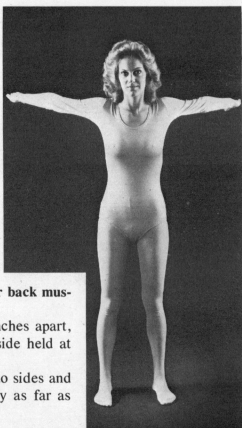

BICEP STRETCH (biceps and upper back muscles)
1. Stand erect with feet about 12 inches apart, arms bent, elbows out to each side held at shoulder height.
2. Slowly extend arms straight out to sides and push them back behind the body as far as possible.
3. Return to starting position.

CROSS-LEGGED TWIST (trunk, shoulder and back muscles)

1. Sit cross-legged on the floor, hands clasped behind neck.
2. Twist your body slowly to the right as far as possible.
3. Return to starting position.
4. Twist your body slowly to the left as far as possible.
5. Return to starting position.

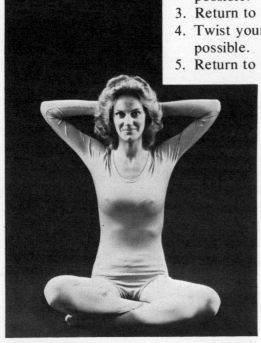

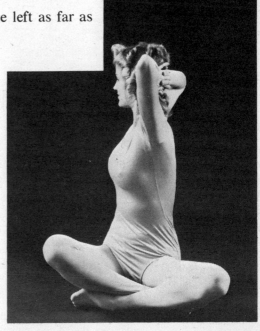

SEATED TOE TOUCHES (lower back and hamstring muscles)

1. Sit on floor, legs extended straight out in front, feet together, arms outstretched in front of body.
2. With toes pointed, bend at waist, trying to touch hands to your toes.
3. To increase stretch, grasp ankles and pull head as close to legs as possible.
4. Return to starting position.

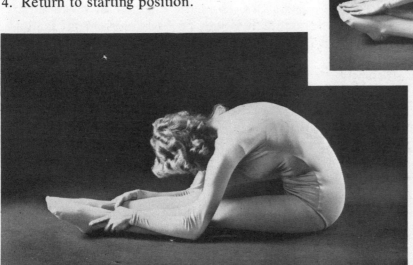

CHAPTER 3

Muscular Strength

MUSCULAR STRENGTH is necessary for any physical accomplishment—from picking up a bag of groceries to developing a strong tennis backhand. Without sufficient strength, your attempts to improve a particular skill—like your tennis backhand—will be hindered and your attempts to improve your flexibility and endurance in a physical fitness program will be limited. Although the fitness elements of flexibility, strength and endurance are all interrelated, it is your muscular system and the demands you put on it that affect development of fitness in the other two elements. If you do not have the abdominal strength to do a situp, you cannot develop endurance in the abdominal muscle group. If you do not have sufficient strength in your lower back muscles, you will find the lower back flexibility exercises difficult if not impossible. Though total physical fitness involves more than strength development, muscular strength is a prerequisite to development of the other conditioning elements.

How much strength you need for everyday tasks and/or participation in a fitness program is difficult to determine. However, a minimum amount of muscle strength is needed to maintain good posture and physique and to efficiently carry out your daily tasks. It's safe to say that if you are not a physically active person—going from home to office and home again with the only exercise being some skiing or football with the kids on the weekends—your strength is at or below minimum. Muscles are meant to be used. When not used or used enough, they begin to deteriorate. This deterioration not only affects your physical appearance—loose, flabby arms, legs and stomach—but also decreases your efficiency. You must use more energy for a given

movement or task than a physically fit person. By increasing your strength, you improve your posture and muscle tone, thus your physical appearance. You can perform heavier tasks in less time with less energy and with more body efficiency. In addition, you run less risk of injuring the major joints in your body and reduce minor aches, stiffness and soreness brought on by everyday tasks. To determine if you have the very minimum strength requirements in your lower back, arm, shoulder and abdominal muscles, go back to the Personal Physical Fitness Evaluation Chart in Chapter 1. If you passed all the Muscular Strength Tests, you possess the *minimum* amount of strength that is considered healthy. If you failed any one or all of the tests, your health could very well be in danger.

METHODS FOR STRENGTH DEVELOPMENT

There are three exercise methods for developing muscle strength—**isometrics, isotonics** and **isokinetics.** Isometric exercise involves muscle contraction with no body movement; isotonic exercise (calisthenics and weight training) refers to muscle contractions with movement; and isokinetic exercise involves muscle contraction with movement and with a controlled resistance. Each of these methods has its advantages and disadvantages.

Isometrics has received much attention largely because strength is developed without any body movement. In performing isometric exercises, a muscle or muscle group is exerted against an immovable object such as a wall or against another muscle group. The chief advantages are that no equipment is needed to perform the exercises and they can be performed anywhere at anytime—sitting behind the desk at the office, in the commuter train, at the theater or standing at the bus stop. Each exercise only takes 6-8 seconds so that the time invested for significant returns in muscle strength is minimal. The non-body movement and brief exercise time make isometrics ideal for the bedridden or wheelchair-confined person or for those people who must spend many of the hours of the day sitting. There is also some evidence that isometric exercise is efficient as a spot reducer, especially in the waist, hip and thigh regions.

However, isometric exercises do have their disadvantages. The most glaring is the fact that for an increase in strength, you must exert two-thirds of your maximum force. In doing an isometric exercise, it's difficult to know if you're exerting enough to make an improvement. You have no definite way of knowing whether you're exerting 10 percent, 50 percent or 100 percent of your force. Another problem is the specificity of isometric exercise. Each exercise is for one muscle area. Because of this, you have to exercise each muscle area for any kind of general conditioning. And this brings up another problem—boredom. In performing a battery of isometric exercises designed for improving each body muscle group, it's easy to lose your concentration because of the sameness and lack of movement. Finally, isometric exercises do absolutely *nothing* for muscular endurance or flexibility. In fact, isometrics without supplementary flexibility exercises can actually reduce the range of movement in your joints.

Isotonic exercises are the two types most of us are most familiar with—*calisthenics* and *weight training*. Calisthenic exercises have several advantages. Very little or no equipment is required for doing the exercises; they're easy to learn and perform; vigorous workouts can be done in short periods of time; you can work on specific areas of the body; and last, very little space is needed for performing the exercises. Unfortunately, calisthenics are the least effective of all the methods for rapid increases in muscle strength. However, for the average adult who wants to develop adequate strength and improve muscle tone, calisthenics will fulfill the need.

It is generally agreed that weight training is the fastest and best method for increasing muscle strength. Weight training is a systematic series of resistance exercises using the overload principle. As the capacity of a muscle or group of muscles increases in strength, the intensity, or weight in the case of weight training, is also increased. Using weight training you can precisely control the exercise load and easily single out and work on a specific muscle or muscle group.

However, there are some disadvantages to weight training. First of all is the cost of the equipment and/or finding a gym to work out in that has all the equipment. Secondly, weight training does not improve cardiovascular fitness and at best should be used as a supplement to flexibility and cardiovascular exercises. In fact, some weight lifting exercises, especially those which require only limited movement, can actually reduce the flexibility in your joints if not supplemented. Even though some might think working with heavy weights might be a disadvantage in that you are risking injury, if the proper precautions are taken with respect to proper breathing, doing the exercises correctly and properly adjusting the weight, injury risk is minimal.

Isokinetic exercises are most widely associated with the exercise machines found in health clubs. These machines control the amount of resistance against which the exerciser works. At a slow speed there is very little resistance but as speed is increased, so is the amount of resistance. Since the machines adapt automatically to the amount of effort being exerted, there is little chance of overstressing a muscle or damaging a weak area such as the knee. Isokinetic machines also allow the exerciser to work on isolated muscle groups with a variety of special exercises. This specific body conditioning is of great benefit to the athlete or sports enthusiast who has special sport technique needs.

Once again, isokinetic exercises do not help build cardiovascular endurance or flexibility and should therefore not be used as a total program but merely as a supplement to build strength and muscle endurance. The other disadvantage is finding the machines to work on. Joining a health club can bite into the pocket a bit. If you have a YMCA or YWCA close by, they may have a Nautlius, Apollo Exerciser or Pro-Gym. If you don't want to join a health club and/or do not have access to any type of isokinetic machine, it is possible to do isokinetic exercises with the help of a partner. The disadvantage of this method is that the resistance which the partner exerts is not nearly as controlled, but nevertheless can be effective. The isokinetic exercises in this chapter will be those which require a partner.

STRENGTH DEVELOPING EXERCISES

How much strength will you develop in doing these exercises? It depends on how much strength you have when you start the exercises. It also depends on your body composition and type. As noted previously, there are notable differences in people's bodies and some will never acquire the strength or musculature that others will, no matter how diligently they work at it.

The person who is already blessed by good muscular development won't come close to seeing the quick improvement that the underdeveloped exerciser will achieve. In some cases, the well-developed person will soon reach the stage where all he accomplishes by strength exercises is maintenance of the strength he already possesses.

The beginner, however, whose musculature is relatively undeveloped will see fast and vast improvements, usually in 3 to 4 weeks. In fairness, it should be said that after that first period of development, gains in strength will come more slowly and won't be nearly so pronounced.

Before getting into the various strength developing exercises, it is important to realize the interrelationship of strength and endurance. When doing exercises to improve your develop-

ment in one, you are going to gain some improvement in the other. However, a minimum amount of strength is needed in order to improve and build up your endurance. All of the calisthenic, weight training and isokinetic exercises in this chapter can be used to build both strength and endurance. It is the way in which you perform the exercise that determines which fitness element you are improving the most.

Strength is the ability of a muscle of muscle group to overcome a maximum resistance in one effort—for example, being able to perform a bicep curl with a 100-pound weight.

Endurance, on the other hand, is the ability of a muscle or muscle group to sustain an effort for a period of time—for example, being able to do 50 bicep curls with a 50-pound weight. A strength developing exercise involves *few* repetitions (usually 6-10) with a maximum amount of resistance, while endurance exercises involve *many* repetitions with a lesser amount of resistance. So in doing the following exercises, the object is not how many repetitions you can perform but how much resistance you can progressively overcome.

For building strength, then, you need to overcome progressively increased resistances. For weight training exercises that means simply adding to the amount of weight you are lifting. For calisthenics, since the only resistance is the weight of your body, you can employ the use of a slant board which increases resistance against the force of gravity or do the exercises using some sort of weight. For the isokinetic exercises, using a partner, simply have the partner apply more resistance.

Isometrics

When performing the following isometric exercises use two-thirds of your maximum force—less than that will be of little benefit. Hold each contraction for 6-8 seconds and during the contraction do little breathing—try to only breathe between contractions. There is no set order for doing the following exercises nor do you have to do them all at one time. But to gain the most benefit from isometrics, the exercises should be done three times during the day. Remember that isometric exercises are very specific so that for general body conditioning, you should pick at least one exercise for each muscle group in the body.

NECK PUSH (neck muscles)

1. Standing or sitting, place the heel of your right hand on your right temple.
2. Push to the right with your head and push to the left with your hand.
3. Hold for 6-8 seconds using two-thirds of your maximum force.
4. Using left hand against left temple, repeat exercise.
5. With hands clasped, place palms of hands on forehead and repeat exercise.
6. With hands clasped, place palms on back of head and repeat exercise.

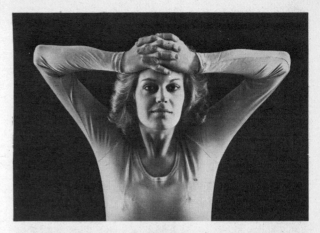

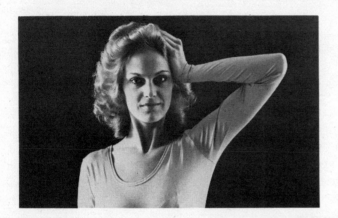

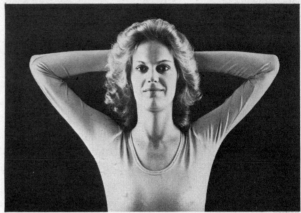

ARM AND SHOULDER PUSH (arm and chest muscles)

1. Stand in doorway and place hands at shoulder height on either side of doorway.
2. Push outward using two-thirds of your maximum force for 6-8 seconds.

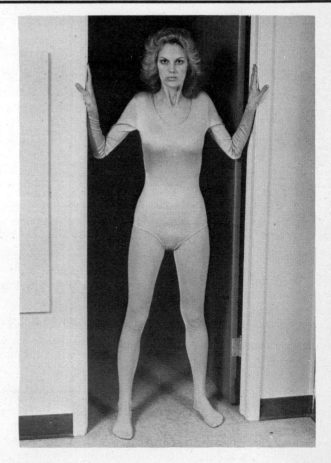

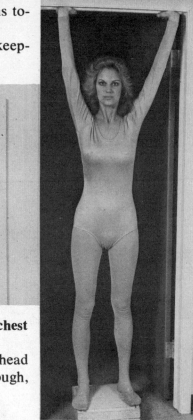

SIDE ARM PUSH (shoulder muscles)
1. Stand in doorway, hands at sides, palms toward legs.
2. Press hands outward against doorway, keeping elbows straight, for 6-8 seconds.

←

→

OVERHEAD PUSH (shoulder, arm and chest muscles)
1. Stand in doorway and place hands overhead on door casing. (If you're not tall enough, stand on a sturdy, hard chair.)
2. Push upwards for 6-8 seconds.

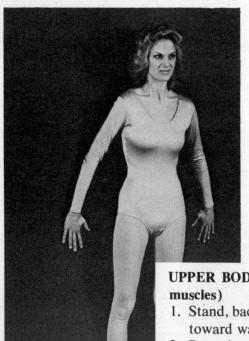

UPPER BODY PUSH (chest, shoulder and arm muscles)
1. Stand, back to the wall, hands at sides, palms toward wall.
2. Press hands backward against wall, keeping arms straight for 6-8 seconds.
3. Reverse position with face to wall, hands at sides, palms toward wall.
4. Press hands forward against wall, keeping arms straight, for 6-8 seconds.

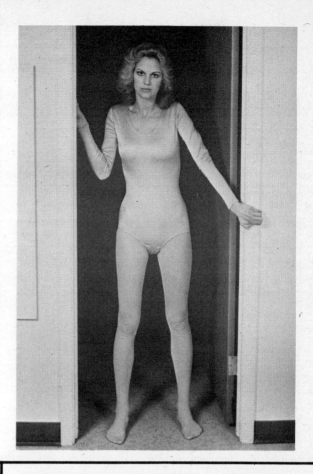

TRUNK PUSH AND PULL (shoulder, arm and trunk muscles)

1. Stand in doorway, legs comfortably apart, with right hand grasping the front of the door casing and the left hand grasping the back of the door casing.
2. Pull with the right hand and push with the left, as if to twist the body to the right against the pressure. Hold for 6-8 seconds.
3. Reverse hand positions with the left hand grasping front of casing and right hand grasping the back of door casing. Try twisting body to the left against pressure for 6-8 seconds.

HAND PULL (triceps and chest muscles)

1. Stand with feet comfortably apart, knees slightly flexed. Grip fingers of both hands, arms close to chest.
2. Pull outward with both arms for 6-8 seconds.

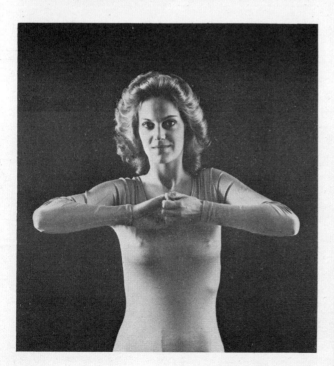

HAND PUSH (biceps and chest muscles)

1. Stand with feet comfortably spaced, knees slightly flexed. Clasp hands, palms together, close to chest.
2. Press hands together for 6-8 seconds.

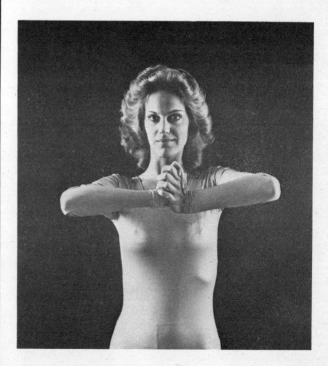

CHAIR LIFT (biceps)

1. Sitting in a chair, feet flat on floor, grip underside of seat with both hands.
2. Pull up for 6-8 seconds.

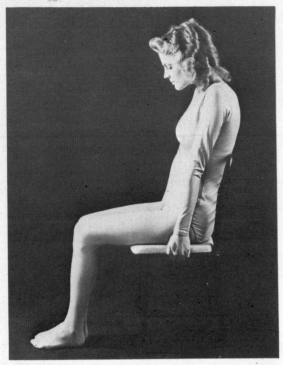

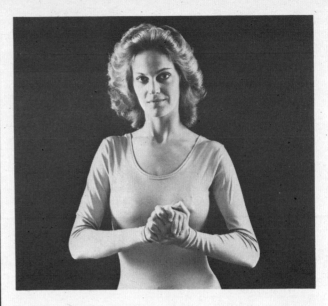

HAND CURL (arm muscles)

1. Stand with feet slightly apart. Flex right elbow, close to body, palm up. Place left hand over right and clasp tightly.
2. Attempt to curl right arm upward toward chest, while giving equally strong resistance with the left hand, for 6-8 seconds.
3. Reverse hand positions and repeat exercise.

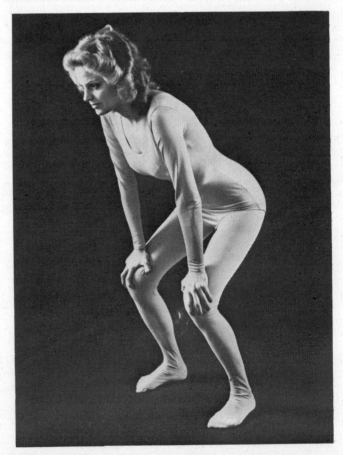

ABDOMINAL SQUEEZE (abdominal muscles)

1. Stand with knees slightly flexed, hands on knees.
2. Contract abdominal muscles for 6-8 seconds.

LOWER BODY PUSH (lower back, buttock and thigh muscles)

1. Lie face down on floor, arms at sides, palms up, legs placed under table, bed or other heavy object.
2. Keeping hips flat on floor, raise right leg, keeping knee straight so that heel pushes against resistance. Push for 6-8 seconds.
3. Repeat exercise pushing for 6-8 seconds with left leg.

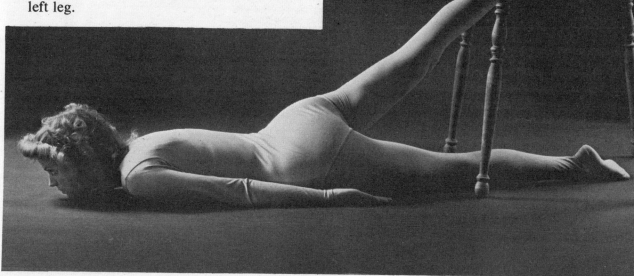

THIGH PUSH (thigh muscles)

1. Sit in chair with feet flat on floor and hands palms down on thighs.
2. Push downward with arms and push upward with thighs for 6-8 seconds.

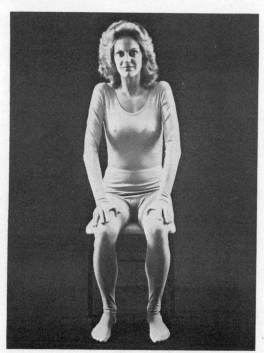

INNER THIGH SQUEEZE (inner thigh muscles)

1. Sit in chair, arms extended, hands closed in fists and fists placed on inside of each knee.
2. Push outward with arms and push inward with thighs for 6-8 seconds.

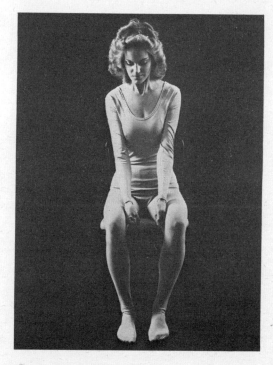

35

RAISED LEG PUSH (leg muscles)

1. Sit in chair, legs extended straight out, right ankle crossed over left ankle, hands gripping sides of chair.
2. Push down with right leg and push up with equal force with left leg for 6-8 seconds.
3. Repeat exercise with reversed leg positions—the left ankle crossed over the right ankle.

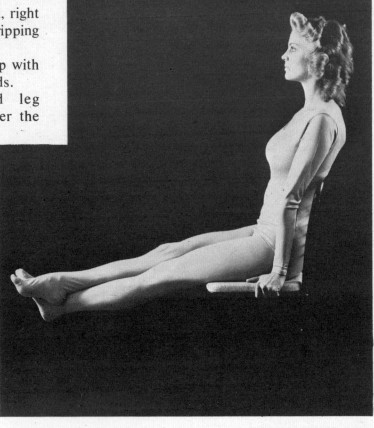

INNER AND OUTER THIGH PUSH (inner and outer thigh muscles)

1. Sit in chair, legs extended with each ankle pressed against the outside of sturdy chair legs.
2. Keeping legs straight, try to pull them together for 6-8 seconds.
3. For outer thigh muscles, place ankles inside the chair legs and push outward for 6-8 seconds.

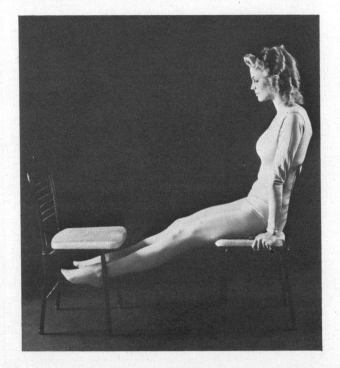

SITTING LEG PUSH AND PULL (leg muscles)

1. Sit in chair with left ankle crossed over right, feet resting on floor, legs bent at 90-degree angle. Hands should be gripping underside of chair.
2. Try to straighten right leg while resisting with left for 6-8 seconds.
3. Reverse leg positions with right ankle crossed over left and repeat exercise.

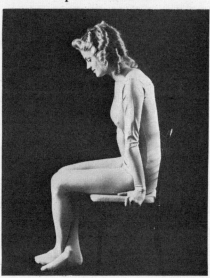

PUSHUP (arm, shoulder and chest muscles)

1. Lie face down on the floor, legs together, hands on floor under shoulders with fingers pointing straight ahead.
2. Push body off floor by extending arms so that your weight rests on hands and toes.
3. Keeping back straight, lower body until chest touches floor.

Calisthenics (Isotonics)

Perhaps the best approach to building strength using calisthenics is the use of circuit training. With this method you choose a sequence of 6-10 calisthenic exercises for the muscles you wish to strengthen. To begin you determine the maximum number of each exercise that you can do in 1 minute. When you've determined this number, reduce it by one-third for each exercise —e.g., if you can do 21 situps in 1 minute, reduce that number by one-third, which would be 14 situps. Once you've reduced your maximum number for each exercise by one-third, your objective is to complete the "circuit" of exercises in a progressively diminishing amount of time. For example, the first time you try completing all the exercises for the predetermined repetitions, it may take you 7 minutes. The next time you may complete the circuit in 6 minutes, so you add 1 repetition to each exercise. For a good 21-minute workout, you should complete three 7-minute circuits. To impose increased demands, the number of repetitions for each exercise is increased while the time remains the same.

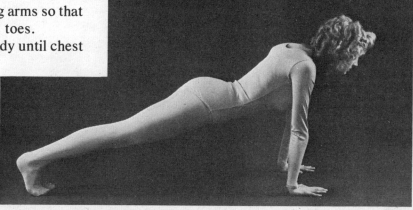

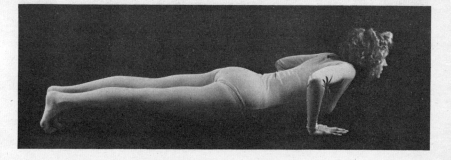

37

CHINUP (arm and shoulder muscles)

1. With chinning bar adjusted to approximately 3 inches beyond extended arm, grasp bar with underhand grip.
2. Flex arms, raising body until chin is over bar.
3. Return to starting position.

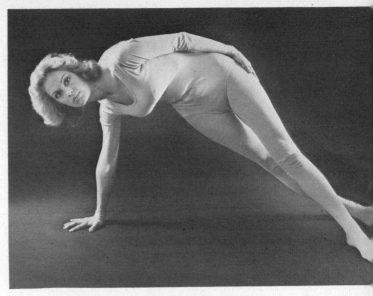

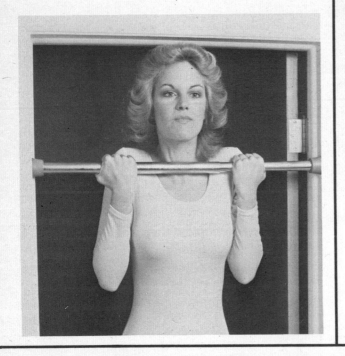

COFFEE GRINDER (arm, shoulder, lateral trunk muscles)

1. Support body on the floor with extended right hand and right foot with left arm at side.
2. Move feet and body in a circle using right arm as a pivot.
3. Repeat exercise with left arm and foot extended.

CHAIR DIP (arm and shoulder muscles)

1. Using a stationary chair, grasp sides of chair, keeping arms straight, sliding feet forward so that your weight rests on your arms.
2. Keeping back straight, lower body as far as possible and return to starting position.

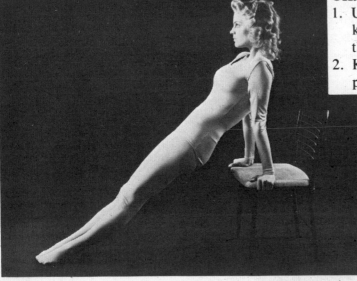

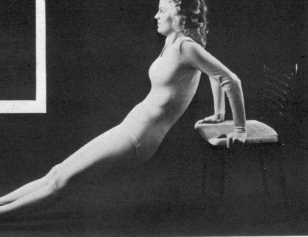

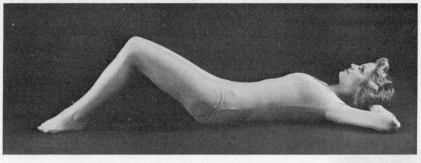

SITUP (abdominal muscles)

1. Lie face up on floor with knees bent and fingers laced behind head.
2. Curl up to sitting position, keeping feet flat on floor and touch right elbow to left knee.
3. Return to starting position and repeat, alternating right and left elbow touches.

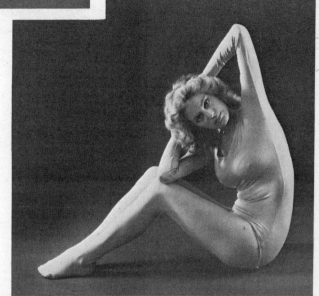

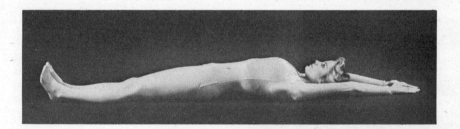

"V" SIT (abdominal muscles)

1. Lie face up on floor, legs straight, arms extended straight behind head.
2. Raise legs and arms up and forward so body forms a "V."
3. Return to starting position.

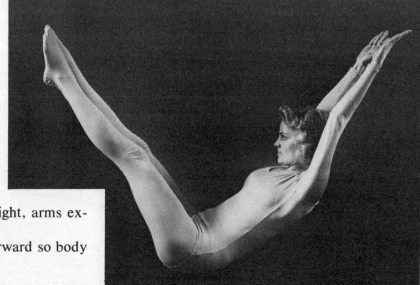

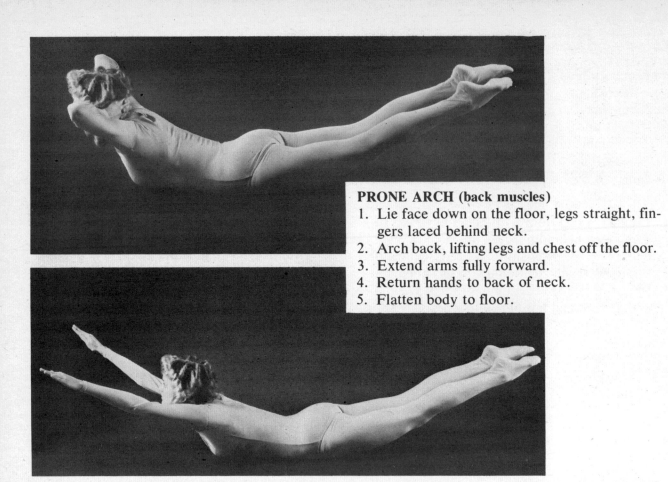

PRONE ARCH (back muscles)
1. Lie face down on the floor, legs straight, fingers laced behind neck.
2. Arch back, lifting legs and chest off the floor.
3. Extend arms fully forward.
4. Return hands to back of neck.
5. Flatten body to floor.

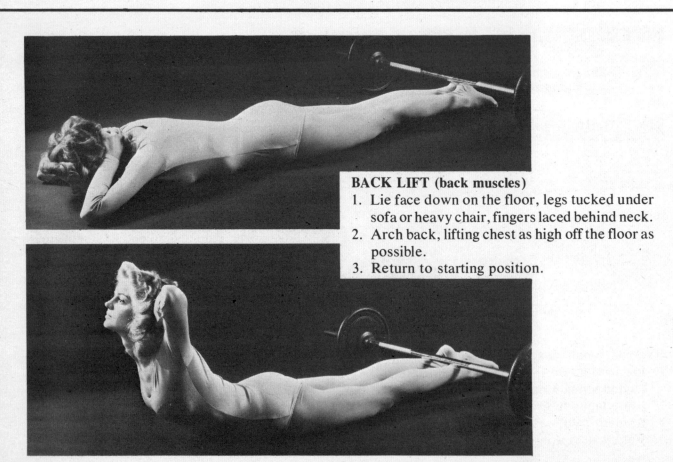

BACK LIFT (back muscles)
1. Lie face down on the floor, legs tucked under sofa or heavy chair, fingers laced behind neck.
2. Arch back, lifting chest as high off the floor as possible.
3. Return to starting position.

Weight Training (Isotonics)

Weight *lifting* is the term used to describe the competitive sport. Weight *training* is a more precise name for exercises used for physical development and conditioning. It is the use of weights combined with the "overload" principle, in which intensity, load and repetition vary according to the individual program. In weight training, a participant never tries to see how much he can lift. Resistance progression is the procedure.

Equipment: Weight training exercises require the use of a weight rack, weight bench, slant board, barbells, dumbbells and a set of variable progressive weights. Barbells are probably the most familiar to us since they are used by weight lifters in weight lifting competition. Barbells vary in length from 4-6 feet with weighted plates of 1¼, 2½, 5, 10 and 25 pounds and more. A sturdy bench has many uses in a weight training program. It should be 6 feet long, 10 inches wide and 20 inches high with an attached weight rack. Though available commercially, the bench can be easily constructed using 2x4's and 3/4-inch plywood with some sort of thick rubber matting for padding the top of the bench. The slant board is also available commercially but can also be constructed easily.

Note: Where possible, two exercises for the same muscle or muscle group are given—one exercise utilizing the barbell, the other dumbbells. In this way, both sets of weight equipment are not necessary to perform the exercises in this section.

Weight Loads: Determining the amount of weight you should start training with is a job of trial and error. One rule-of-thumb is to start with 10 pounds less than you think you can lift. A better way is to systematically test each muscle group by the trial and error method. As mentioned previously, for maximum strength gain, no less than six and no more than ten repetitions should be done for each exercise. To determine the correct weight load to start out with, you must experiment for each muscle group to find out the amount of weight which allows the repetitions to remain within that range. For example, to test your biceps, you attempt to do six to ten bicep curls with a 50-pound weight. If you can complete only five curls, you must reduce the weight by 20 percent or 10 pounds and try the test again. If, on the second test, you completed eight curls with the 50-pound weight, then that is the weight you should start with. If, for the first test, you could do 12 bicep curls with the 50-pound weight, then, the weight is too light and should be increased by 20 percent or 10 pounds. Although this may seem time consuming, resist the temptation to "see how much I can lift." This trial and error method will allow you to determine *safely* the amount of weight that will afford you the greatest gains in strength development and will keep you safe from muscle or joint strains which could result from lifting more than your body can handle. Remember that each joint and muscle group in your body has its own specific weight tolerances—so a determination of weight amount for one muscle group is not applicable to another.

Principles and Safety Factors: The following principles and safety factors should be implemented in any weight training program.

1. Never hold your breath during a lift. This can cause an increase in blood pressure, overwork the heart and restrict the return of blood to the heart and arteries. Exhale during the lift and inhale as the weight is lowered.
2. When lifting heavy weight loads, work with a companion or "spotter" who is ready to assist in case anything should go wrong.
3. The starting poundage should not cause any undue strain. As previously advised, use the trial and error system for determining starting weight and progress to heavier loads.
4. Each exercise should be performed rhythmically and through the full range of joint motion for the joint being exercised. (For some of the weight lifting exercises, it is not possible to perform the exercise through the full range of joint motion. Flexibility exercises should be done to maintain mobility in the joint.) Performing exercises with weights in a jerky fashion can be dangerous, resulting in joint or muscle injury.
5. A weight training session should be preceded by a warm-up and followed by a cooling-off period.
6. Check your equipment before lifting. A loose collar could result in weight plates falling off and injury to the lifter.
7. *NEVER* attempt to dead lift weights off the

floor with knees locked in the extended position and the trunk of your body at a 90-degree angle to the floor. This is almost certain injury to your back. The proper stance is with feet parallel and shoulder width apart, your toes as close to the bar as possible, your hips lowered by flexing the knees, the head looking straight forward, and your back straight.

8. If you want to develop power, you do it by reducing the total weight and increasing the speed of the full motion of an exercise. You develop endurance by reducing the total weight and doing the exercise more times at a slower speed.

9. An alternate day, 3-day-a-week weight training program is all that is necessary for strength development.

Weight Training for Women: One myth surrounding weight training is that a woman who lifts weights for strength development and physique improvement will acquire the large musculature of a man. This is simply not true. It is physically impossible for a woman to develop muscle masses comparable to those of a man. First of all, women lack enough of the hormone androgen, which is the primary factor responsible for male's muscles' massive response to weight training. Secondly, a woman's muscles are surrounded by much more adipose tissue (fat) than those of a man. When a man trains with weights, the amount of fat between the skin and the muscle rapidly disappears with the skin stretched tightly exposing the large muscle. When a woman trains with weights, a small percentage of this same adipose disappears but enough remains so the muscle is not exposed. Finally, a woman's muscles are much smaller than a man's, thus no amount of weight training is going to make a woman muscle-bound. So women who were going to skip over this portion of the book—don't. Working with weights will do wonders for your muscle tone and body shape.

SITUP (abdominal muscles)
Equipment: dumbbell or weight plate
1. Lie face up on the floor, feet tucked under a couch or heavy chair, knees flexed, hands holding a dumbbell or weight plate behind neck.
2. Curl up into sitting position, touching elbows to knees.
3. Return to starting position to repeat.
Note: For increased resistance without weight change, do this same exercise on a slant board with toes strapped to top of board and head at bottom.

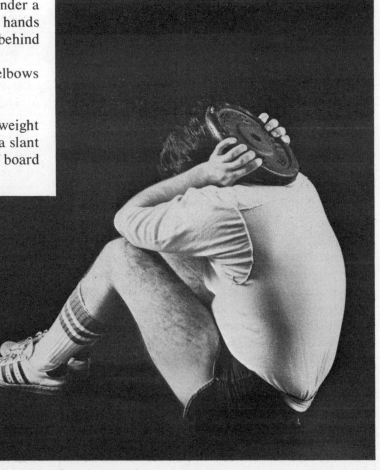

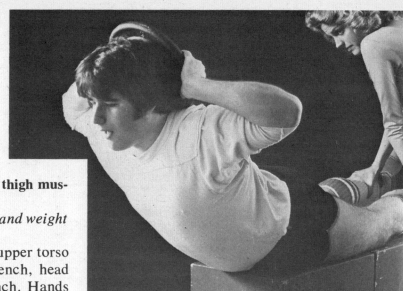

TRUNK RAISE (lower back, hip and thigh muscles)

Equipment: dumbbell or weight plate and weight bench or table

1. Lie face down on the bench with upper torso extending over the end of the bench, head toward floor. Strap ankles to bench. Hands hold the dumbbell or weight plate behind the neck.
2. Lift upper body to parallel position with the floor but no higher.
3. Return to starting position to repeat.

HEEL RAISE (calf muscles)

Equipment: barbell with towel wrapped around bar, block of wood 2 inches thick, barbell racks or spotter

1. Stand with toweled portion of barbell against back of neck, hands gripping bar in overhand grip, knees flexed, feet 6-10 inches apart, toes on block of wood.
2. Straighten knees and lift heels as high as possible above block of wood.
3. Return heels to floor.

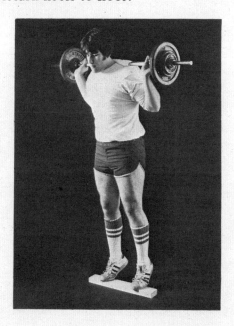

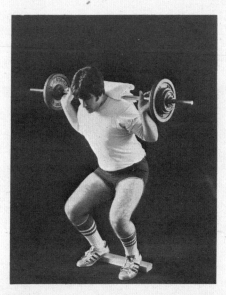

HALF KNEE BENDS (hip, ankle and thigh muscles)

Equipment: barbell with towel wrapped around bar, block of wood 2 inches thick, barbell racks or spotter

1. Stand with toweled portion of barbell against back of neck, hands gripping bar in overhand grip, knees flexed, feet 8-10 inches apart, toes on floor, heels on block of wood.
2. Squat slightly as shown but no further because of possible injury to knee joint.
3. Return to starting position to repeat.

SQUAT STAND (hip, ankle and thigh muscles)

Equipment: barbell

1. Stand straddling barbell with barbell at 90-degree angle to body.
2. Bend at knees and waist, keeping back straight and grip barbell with one hand at rear and the other at front.
3. Straighten knees slowly until fully extended, lifting weight off floor.
4. Bend at the knees to lower barbell but do not let it touch the floor to repeat.

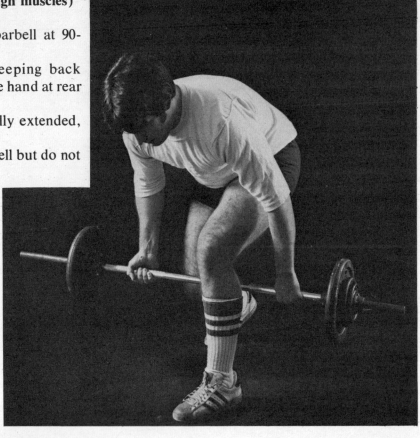

ARM RAISE (arm biceps and deltoids and chest muscles)

Equipment: weight bench and dumbbells

1. Lie face up on bench with knees over end of bench, feet flat on floor, arms fully extended above body, each hand gripping a dumbbell.
2. Slowly lower arms toward floor as far as possible. (It may be necessary to bend elbows slightly to stabilize elbow joint.)
3. Raise arms slowly to starting position.

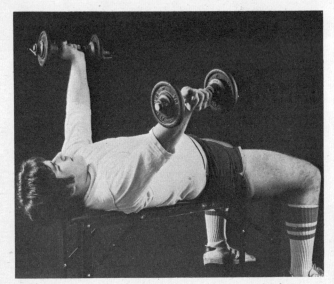

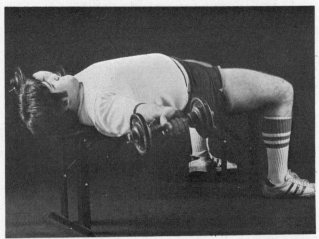

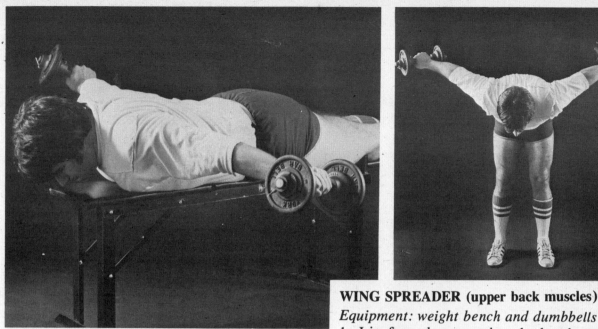

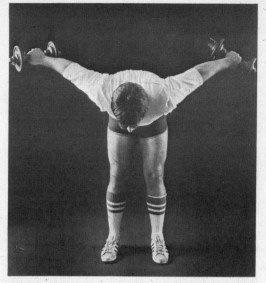

WING SPREADER (upper back muscles)
Equipment: weight bench and dumbbells
1. Lie face down on bench, hands gripping dumbbells on floor.
2. Raise dumbbells to shoulder height.
3. Lower dumbbells to floor.
Note: This exercise can be done in standing position with feet slightly apart and upper trunk parallel to floor.

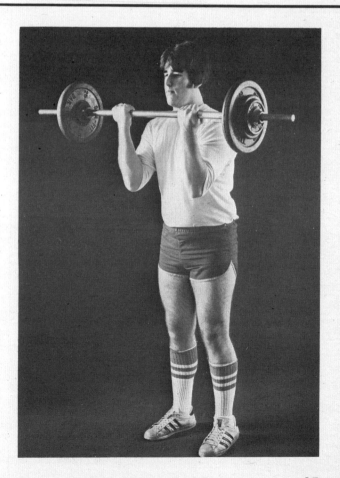

BICEPS CURL (bicep muscles)
Equipment: barbell
1. Stand erect, feet comfortably apart, knees slightly flexed. With arms slightly flexed at elbows, hold barbell in front of you with underhand grip, hands shoulder width apart.
2. Flex elbows fully, lifting bar to chest, keeping elbows close to sides. (*Don't* lean backward or "bounce" bar with leg motion.)
3. Return to starting position to repeat.

TRICEPS EXTENSION (tricep muscles)

Equipment: weight bench and barbell

1. Sit astride bench with back straight, hands gripping bar in overhand grip.
2. Raise bar above head.
3. Lower bar behind head by bending elbows.
4. Raise arms to full arm extension to repeat.

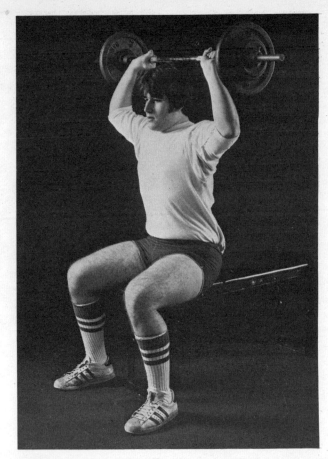

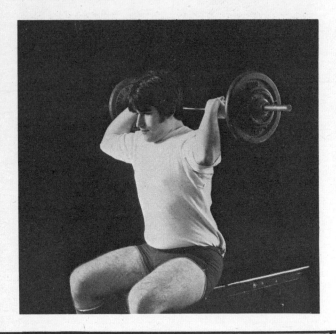

OVERHEAD ARM RAISE (tricep muscles)

Equipment: dumbbells

1. Stand erect, feet comfortably apart, arm straight overhead, gripping dumbbell.
2. Lower forearm by bending elbow behind head, keeping upper arm stationary.
3. Raise arm to full extension to repeat.
4. Repeat exercise with opposite arm.

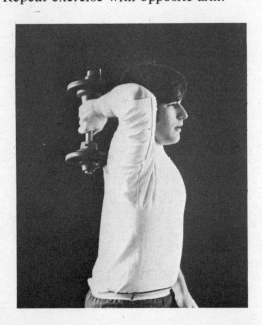

HIGH PULL (shoulder muscles)

Equipment: barbell

1. Stand erect, feet comfortably apart, hands gripping barbell in overhand grip, the weight held just below waist.
2. Bend elbows and raise weight straight up to chin level.
3. Return to starting position to repeat.

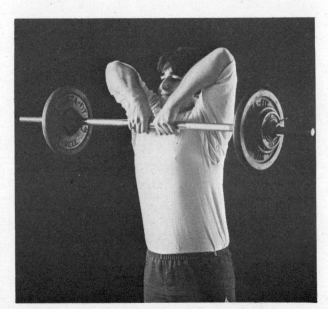

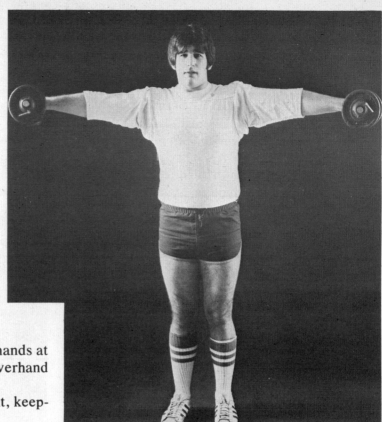

SIDE ARM RAISE (shoulder muscles)
Equipment: dumbbell
1. Stand erect, feet comfortably apart, hands at sides, each gripping dumbbell in overhand grip.
2. Raise arms laterally to shoulder height, keeping elbows straight.
3. Return to starting position to repeat.

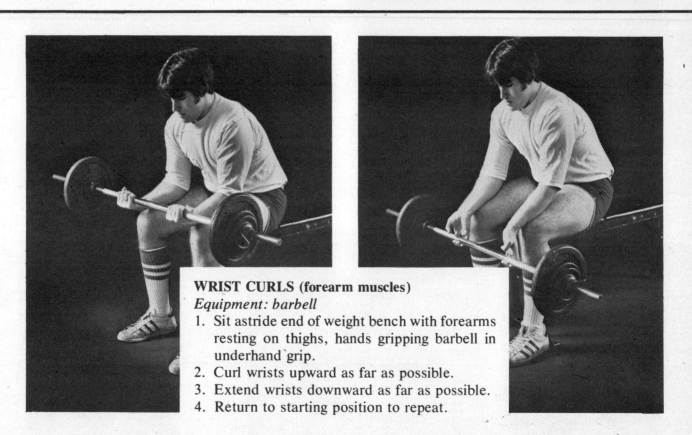

WRIST CURLS (forearm muscles)
Equipment: barbell
1. Sit astride end of weight bench with forearms resting on thighs, hands gripping barbell in underhand grip.
2. Curl wrists upward as far as possible.
3. Extend wrists downward as far as possible.
4. Return to starting position to repeat.

FOREARM RAISE (thumb side muscles of forearm)

Equipment: dumbbell with only one end weighted

1. Stand erect, hands at sides, one hand gripping unweighted end of dumbbell in thumb-up grip with weight pointing forward.
2. Raise dumbbell as far as possible without moving forearm.
3. Return to starting position to repeat.
4. Repeat exercise with other arm.

BACK ARM RAISE (little finger side muscles of forearm)

Equipment: dumbbell with only one end weighted

1. Stand erect, hands at sides, one hand gripping unweighted end of dumbbell in thumb-down grip with weight pointing backward.
2. Raise dumbbell as far as possible without moving forearm.
3. Return to starting position to repeat.
4. Repeat exercise with other arm.

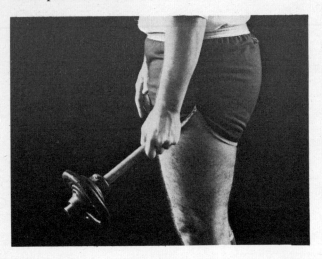
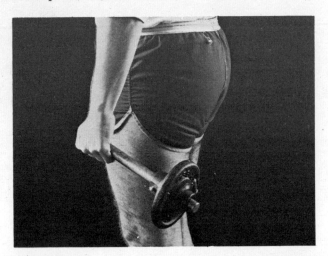

NECK RAISE (neck muscles)

Equipment: weight plate, weight bench and towel

1. Lie face up on bench with head hanging over the end of the bench.
2. Place folded towel on forehead and place weight on top of towel.
3. Raise head as far as possible holding weight stable with hands.
4. Return to starting position to repeat.

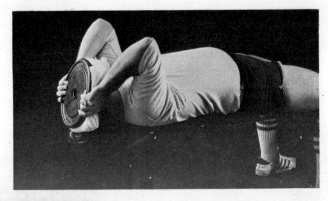
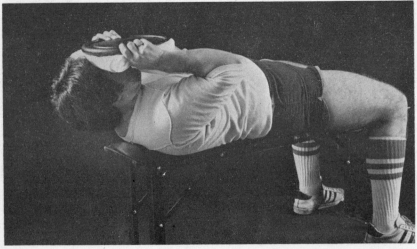

Isokinetics

The isokinetic exercises presented here are ones that can be done with a partner. For those of you who don't want to spend the money on weights but can easily find a workout partner, these exercises are ideal. Each exercise should be done slowly and smoothly with no jerky movement. Through trial and error, you and your partner can work out the amount of resistance that is required.

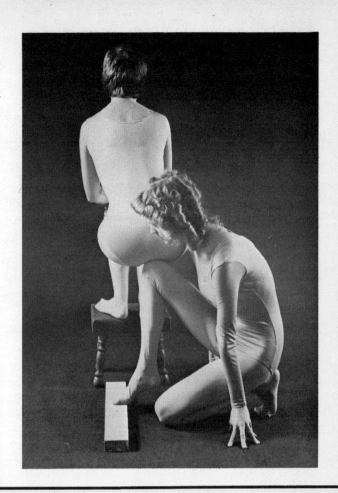

HEEL RAISES (calf muscles)

1. The exerciser kneels on one leg while one toe of other leg rests on 2-inch thick block of wood with heel on floor. Partner sits on knee with feet resting on a bench, couch or similar structure.
2. Exerciser raises heel as far up as possible.
3. Return to starting position to repeat.
4. Repeat exercise with opposite leg.

LEG CURL (hamstring muscles)

1. Lie face down on the floor, knees bent at 90-degree angle to body, feet together, hands at sides.
2. Partner grips your ankles and provides resistance while you curl your heels back toward your back.
3. Return to starting position.

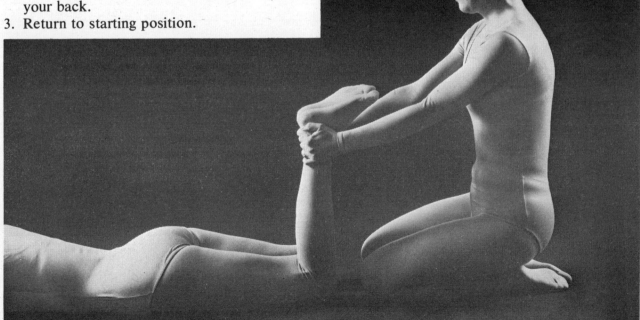

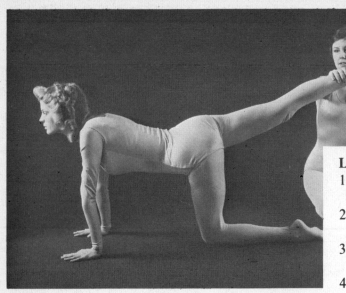

LEG RAISE (buttock muscles)

1. Get down on hands and knees and raise left leg parallel to floor.
2. While partner provides resistance, raise leg above a position parallel with the floor.
3. Return to starting position and raise right leg parallel to floor.
4. Repeat exercise with right leg.

PEC POPPER (chest muscles)

1. Lie face up on floor, left arm at side, right arm extended laterally.
2. While partner provides resistance, raise arm in an arc with your shoulder as the axis point. Bend your elbow only slightly and keep arm moving until your fist is above opposite shoulder.
3. Repeat exercise with left arm.

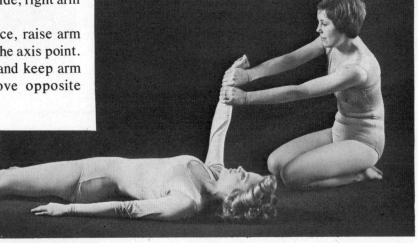

SIDE ARM RAISE (shoulder muscles)

1. Stand erect, feet spread comfortably apart, hands at sides.
2. While partner provides resistance, raise one arm out to the side and up over head, bending elbow only slightly.
3. Repeat exercise with other arm.

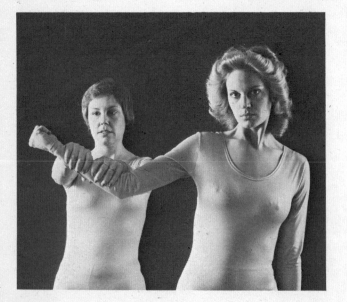

SIDE BEND (trunk muscles)

1. Stand with feet comfortably apart, trunk bent sideways to the right as far as possible, right arm gripped by partner's hands and left arm bent over your head.
2. While your partner provides resistance, try to straighten to upright position.
3. Reverse position to left side and repeat exercise.

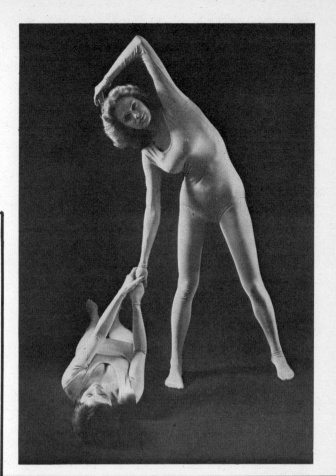

NECK PULL (front neck muscles)

1. Stand erect, feet spread comfortably apart, hands on hips, head bent backward, as far as possible.
2. Partner clasps hands around your forehead and applies resistance while you pull your head forward until chin rests on chest.

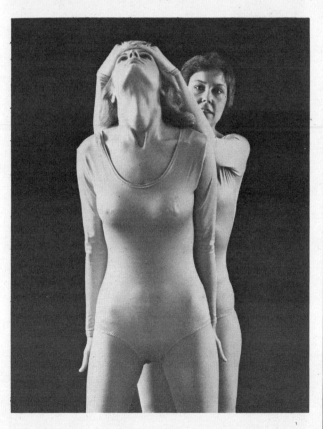

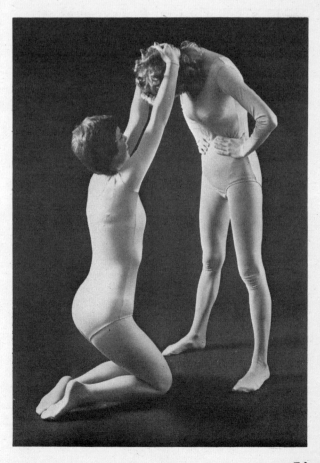

WHIPLASH (rear neck muscles)

1. Stand erect, back to wall or other support, feet spread comfortably apart, hands on hips, head bent forward, chin resting on chest.
2. Partner clasps hands behind your head and provides resistance while you pull your head backward as far as possible.

ARM CURL (biceps and forearm muscles)
1. Stand erect, feet comfortably apart, elbows bent slightly.
2. Partner stands facing you and interlocks his hands with yours—your hands palms up, his palms down.
3. While partner provides resistance, raise your arms to chest by bending elbows.

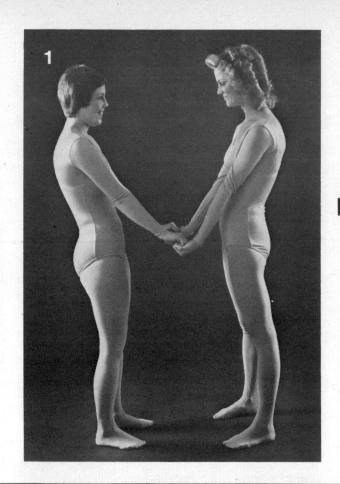

ARM EXTENSION (rear forearm muscles)
1. Stand erect, feet comfortably apart, arms bent at elbows, fists chest high.
2. Partner stands facing you and interlocks his hands with yours—your hands palms down, his palms up.
3. While partner provides resistance, lower arms to sides by bending elbows.

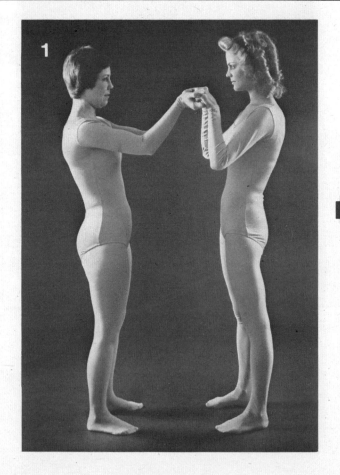

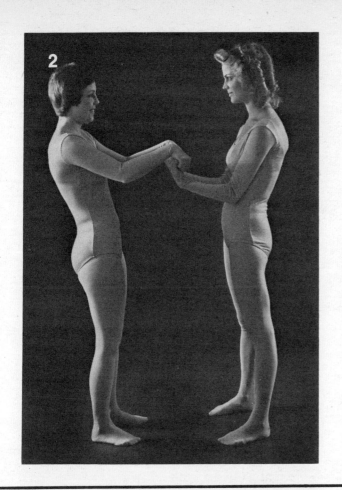

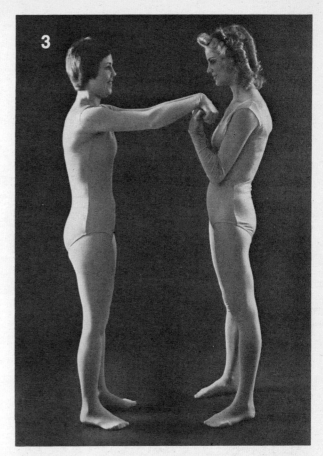

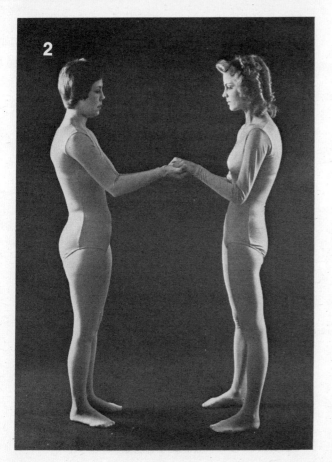

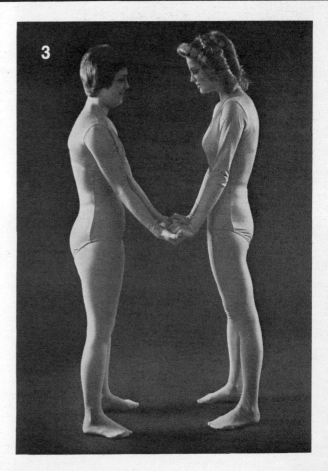

PUSHUP (arm and shoulder muscles)

1. Lie face down on floor, palms on floor under shoulders, feet straight out behind you with toes on floor.
2. Partner stands facing you with hands on shoulders.
3. While partner provides resistance, extend arms, pushing body off floor, keeping back straight, supporting weight on arms and toes.

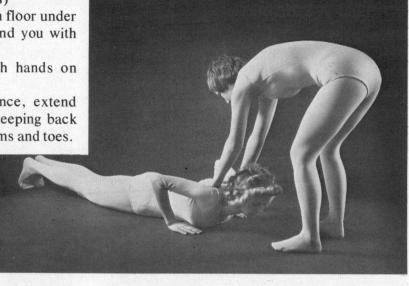

LEG EXTENSION (leg muscles)

1. Sit on table or bench (high enough so feet are off the floor), hands gripping sides of table.
2. Partner stands facing you with hands gripping right leg.
3. As partner provides resistance, raise leg parallel to floor.
4. Repeat exercise with left leg.

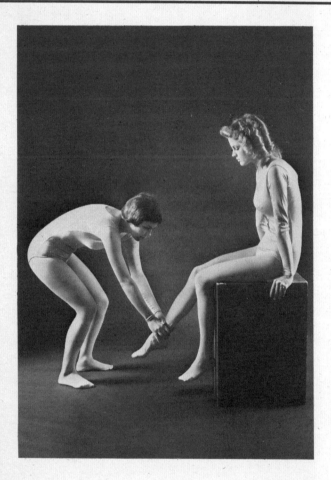

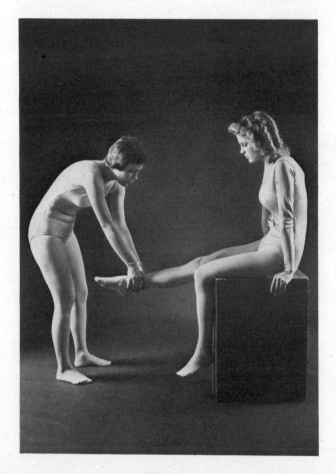

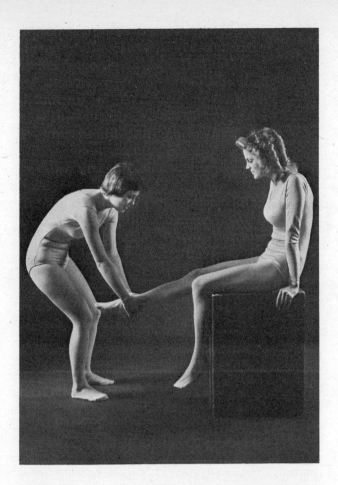

LEG FLEXION (leg muscles)

1. Sit on table or bench (high enough so feet are off the floor), hands gripping sides of table, right leg parallel with floor.
2. Partner stands facing you with hands gripping right leg.
3. As partner provides resistance, lower leg to 90-degree angle.
4. Repeat exercise with left leg.

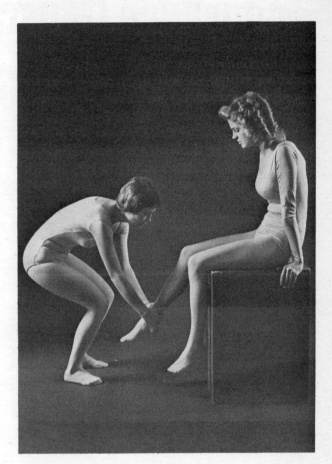

Once you've developed a reasonable amount of strength, you're ready to proceed to the fitness element that is, in our opinion, the most important of all—cardiovascular-pulmonary endurance. If you don't move ahead into it and are content to go no further than the development of strength, you're cheating yourself. With all the pressures of today's world, endurance is the most important physical attribute you can develop.

CHAPTER 4

Endurance (Muscular, Heart-Lung)

ENDURANCE, to put it simply, is the capacity to sustain intense activity for a period of time without excessive fatigue. Endurance is measured by the length of time a muscle or muscle group can sustain a type of activity—for example, how many times a person can repeat an exercise such as situps or pushups, or how long or how far a person can run, swim, or bicycle. Two types of muscle systems are involved in endurance training—*skeletal* and *cardiovascular*. Your skeletal muscles are those needed for movement—neck, arm, trunk and leg muscles. The cardiovascular muscle system includes your heart, lungs and circulatory system. The two muscle systems are interrelated—exercises to improve endurance of one system put demands on the other. However, the exercise methods most effective in building the endurance fitness of the two systems are quite different in nature. To build endurance of the skeletal muscles exercises such as situps, pushups (calisthenics) or bicep curls and bench presses (weight training) are implemented. Dynamic exercises—running, jogging, bicycling, walking or rope jumping (aerobics)—are the only exercises which effectively improve cardiovascular endurance. It is important to realize that to perform a dynamic exercise, such as jogging, you must develop a certain endurance fitness level in your leg, back and abdominal muscles or jogging for long distances becomes impossible. The same holds true for exercises to improve endurance of the skeletal muscles. A certain level of cardiovascular fitness is necessary to do a prolonged series of situps or pushups because of the demands placed upon your heart and circulatory system.

Why do you need to develop endurance? Endurance improves your efficiency and therefore productivity. As your endurance fitness level improves, the energy required to perform a given amount of work decreases. You can perform a task longer with less fatigue. Raking leaves, gardening, painting your house, playing touch football with the kids, tennis, racquetball, even your chosen occupation all demand a certain amount of endurance. A typist, for example, must have enough arm, shoulder and back muscle endurance to type 8 hours a day. A construction worker needs a high degree of endurance to sustain his vigorous work level for 8 hours a day. Even the top executive needs to maintain a certain level endurance.

How do you know whether or not you need to improve your muscular and/or cardiovascular endurance? Ask yourself these questions:

1. Do I tire during the work day?
2. Am I tired at the end of the work day?
3. Do I have enough energy left over after work for hobbies or other leisure-time pursuits?
4. Do I have the energy for weekend chores and some left over for fun or sports activities?

If you seem to tire easily without good reason, if you seem to need lots of naps, if you lack the energy to join the kids or friends in an active game, you need to improve your endurance.

SKELETAL MUSCLE ENDURANCE

Before you attempt to improve the endurance of a specific muscle or muscle group, you must possess adequate strength. Review your scores on the Strength Test in Chapter 1. If you failed any part of the test, you should do exercises to build your muscle strength in that area. Muscle strength is a prerequisite for endurance exercises.

The calisthenic, weight training and isokinetic strength building exercises described in Chapter 3 are also used to build muscular endurance. The main difference between exercising for strength and for endurance is in the number of repetitions. Muscle endurance is developed when a muscle or muscle group works against a light resistance with many repetitions. Strength exercises involve heavy resistance with few repetitions. Endurance exercises should be done at about a rate of 30 per minute. If you are exhausted prior to the 1-minute goal, the resistance or work load is too heavy and you're building strength instead of endurance. If, on the other hand, you are not exhausted at the end of 1 minute and could exercise longer, the resistance is too light and should be increased.

Using the weight training exercises to build endurance, you decrease the amount of resistance and increase the number of repetitions. For example, if you can do 6-10 situps holding a 20-pound weight, reduce the weight to 5 pounds and attempt to do 30 situps in 1 minute. If you are not exhausted at the end of the minute, increase the amount of weight and/or the number of repetitions and the allotted time. By doing this, you are employing the overload principle—as the endurance capacity of a muscle or muscle group increases, the intensity of the exercise is also increased. If you prefer to use calisthenics or isokinetic exercises to increase endurance, do the maximum number of repetitions possible, still using the 30-per-minute rate, rest and then repeat. Always strive to increase the number of repetitions.

Unlike strength exercising, where a 50 percent gain in strength is difficult to attain, muscle endurance gains are many times dramatic. After a few weeks, it is possible to triple or quadruple the number of repetitions of a particular exercise.

CARDIOVASCULAR ENDURANCE

Cardiovascular-pulmonary endurance is the most important aspect of any total physical fitness program. Exercise helps your heart, lungs and circulatory system to perform more efficiently—more work with less effort. With the proper exercise, your heart, which is muscle tissue, increases in strength and can pump more blood through your system in fewer beats per minute, whether you are at rest or engaged in physical activity. For example, the heart of an unconditioned person may pump only 70 percent of the blood in each heart chamber, whereas the heart of a physically fit person may pump 80-90 percent. The heart of the conditioned person doesn't have to work as hard (beats less often) to supply the body with blood. This increase in efficiency enables your heart to respond more effectively and safely to a sudden demand.

In addition to strengthening your heart and improving its efficiency, exercise also improves your ability to take in, transport and utilize oxygen. This is known as aerobic capacity. Your respiratory system becomes more efficient—taking in more air with each breath, thus getting more oxygen into the blood. The increased efficiency of your circulatory system—arteries, capillaries, blood vessels—better distributes blood throughout the body. Increased heart output plus improved distribution leads to an improved supply of oxygen to the muscles. The muscles, which need oxygen to sustain intense activity, can then better respond to long periods of exercise without excessive fatigue.

There is only one exercise method which will efficiently build your cardiovascular-pulmonary endurance—**aerobics.** Aerobic exercise includes *running* and/or *jogging, bicycling, swimming, walking, running in place* or *jumping rope.* They are all dynamic rhythmical activities which will cause a *sustained* increase in heart rate, respiration and muscle metabolism. A sustained exercise will increase the strength and endurance of your heart, lungs and circulatory system and can also reduce body weight by burning a large number of calories in a short period of time.

To benefit from any of the aerobic exercises, the *intensity, duration* and *frequency* of the exercise must be sustained and maintained. The proper intensity is best indicated by the heart beat rate you sustain throughout the exercise period. The intensity of your exercise should be based upon your training heart rate. (See Chapter 1, page 12, to determine your proper training heart rate.) You must increase your heart beat rate to its training rate and then sustain that rate for at least 15 minutes before you can benefit from any aerobic exercise.

To determine if your heart rate has reached the training rate, do 5 minutes of aerobic exercise and then immediately take your pulse for 15 seconds. Multiply that number by four. If your heart rate is below that suggested, you should pick up the pace of your exercise—i.e., if bicycling, pedal at a faster pace. If your heart rate is higher than suggested, slow down your exercise pace. If your heart beat rate is 30 beats *over* the suggested training rate, you have reached your *maximum* heart beat rate. *Slow* down your exercise pace. Take another count after another 5 minutes of exercise to see if you are within your training heart beat range. You should not overstress your heart.

The duration of exercise can be expressed in time, distance or the number of calories burned. We've already stated that an aerobic exercise should be sustained for a minimum of 15 minutes in order to build cardiovascular strength and endurance. In terms of calories, it is recommended that if you rated poor on the Step Test in Chapter 1, your aerobic exercise should last long enough to burn 100 to 200 calories; if you rated average, 200 to 400 calories; and if you rated excellent, you should burn more than 400 calories. To see how many minutes of aerobic exercise it takes to burn 200 calories, see the chart at right.

How frequently should you engage in an aerobic exercise period? For beginners, two or three times a week is enough. As you progress, you can begin to exercise more; the more frequently you exercise, the more progress you make toward fitness. As you can see from the Aerobic Fitness Prescription Chart below, those who rate average or excellent should exercise 6 days a week.

AEROBIC FITNESS PRESCRIPTIONS

Fitness Category		Intensity (in beats/min)	Duration (in calories) Men	Women*	Frequency
Excellent			Over 400†	Over 300†	6 days weekly
	Age 20	164-178			
	25	162-176			
	30	160-174			
	35	157-171	— Exercise duration and frequency		➡
	40	154-168	remain the same regardless of age —		
	45	151-164			
	50	148-161			
	55	145-158			
	60	143-155			
Average			200-400	150-300	6 days weekly
	Age 20	153-164			
	25	151-162			
	30	148-159			
	35	145-157			
	40	142-154	— Exercise duration and frequency		➡
	45	139-151	remain the same regardless of age —		
	50	136-149			
	55	133-146			
	60	130-143			
Poor			100-200	75-150	Every other day
	Age 20	140-154			
	25	137-151			
	30	134-148			
	35	130-144			
	40	126-140	— Exercise duration and frequency		➡
	45	122-136	remain the same regardless of age —		
	50	118-132			
	55	114-128			
	60	110-124			

*Caloric expenditure is less for women, because they are smaller than men and burn fewer calories in a given activity.

†For long duration workouts (over 400 calories), training intensity may be reduced to a comfortable level.

AEROBICS & CALORIES

	Calories per minute*	Time taken to burn approx. 200 calories (in minutes)
Calisthenics	5.0	40
Walking (3½ mph)	5.6	36
Cycling (10 mph)	8.5	24
Swimming (crawl)	9.0	22
Skipping Rope (120/min)	10.0	20
Jogging (5 mph)	10.0	20
Running (7.5 mph)	15.0	14

*Exact calories burned depends on efficiency and body size.

Now that you know how aerobic exercise will benefit your cardiovascular system and how long and how frequently you must participate in aerobic activity, your next decision is which aerobic exercise you will engage in to achieve cardiovascular fitness. First of all, consider your body type, which was discussed in Chapter 1. For each type of body, exercises were given which best suited each body type (see page 11). This may influence your decision on which type of aerobic exercise you choose. But more importantly, you should choose an exercise that you enjoy. If you select an exercise you don't particularly have fun doing, you're not going to stay on a physical fitness program for long.

We'll try to help in your decision by looking at each of the aerobic exercises—when, where and how to do each and what equipment you need in order to participate in each.

AEROBIC ACTIVITIES

Run		Jog		Bicycle		Swim		Walk	
Distance (miles)	Time (min)	Distance (miles)	Time (min)	Distance (miles)	Time (min)	Distance (yd)	Time (min)	Distance (miles)	Time (min)
3.4+	27+	3.4+	40+	7.8+	47+	1,600+	45+	4.2+	72+

— Distance and time remain the same regardless of age —

Run		Jog		Bicycle		Swim		Walk	
1.7-3.4	14-27	1.7-3.4	20-40	3.9-7.8	24-47	800-1,600	22-45	2.1-4.2	36-72

— Distance and time remain the same regardless of age —

Run		Jog		Bicycle		Swim		Walk	
0.8-1.7	7-14	0.8-1.7	10-20	1.9-3.9	12-24	400-800	11-22	1.0-2.1	18-36

— Distance and time remain the same regardless of age —

RUNNING AND JOGGING

Running is the most instinctive form of cardiovascular-pulmonary endurance exercise known to man. Primitive man didn't even know what cardiovascular-pulmonary endurance was. He ran not for that reason but to flee from danger. Even the early American Indians did a lot of running, as couriers and in chasing wild game. Here again, their continued welfare and sometimes their lives depended on the ability to run.

They didn't think about it—they just did it.

Savage tribes in Africa often saved their lives by running away from an enemy that had them outnumbered. Running from danger was the natural thing to do.

And all of these early people had tremendous cardiovascular-pulmonary endurance. When they died, it was rarely from a heart attack but usually from lack of medication for diseases, from an imbalance in diet or from battle wounds. Today in our automated society, few Americans

A SAMPLE AEROBIC TRAINING SESSION

Warm-up, aerobic exercise, cooldown—those are the elements of your training session. Let's look closer at a typical session, say for a 35-year-old man with a fitness evaluation of average, and see how it leads to fitness.

His fitness prescription would be: **intensity,** 145 to 157 beats a minute; **duration,** 200 to 400 calories; **frequency,** every other day at the beginning, then 5 or 6 days a week with 1 day off for good behavior. He has picked jogging as his aerobic exercise. After his warm-up he will jog at a 12-minute-per-mile pace for 20 minutes (1.67 miles) to burn 200 calories (20 minutes at 10 calories a minute). He can vary his sessions by jogging in different locales, working at the upper edge of his training zone for shorter duration, or at the lower edge for longer. After his run, he will cool down with easy jogging, walking and stretching. It won't take too many sessions like this before he begins to experience a *training effect*.

Heart and lungs improve as the body adjusts to regular exercise, and he will soon be able to complete his session at a lower heart rate. As this happens, it's necessary to do something to insure a continued training effect. In the case of our 35-year-old jogger, he could: (1) jog the same distance at a faster pace (but calories burned remain the same); (2) cover a greater distance at the same pace (calories burned increase but intensity falls *below* training zone); (3) slowly increase both pace and distance, thereby keeping heart rate in training zone while increasing calories burned.

In practice, #3 usually occurs naturally. You increase pace without knowing it. You find yourself running faster without a greater sense of effort or fatigue. As fitness improves, it becomes easy to extend the duration of a workout. When you find this happening, you're ready to increase the intensity, duration, and frequency of your training sessions; or periodically retake the Step Test or run the 1½ miles for time to pinpoint your fitness level.

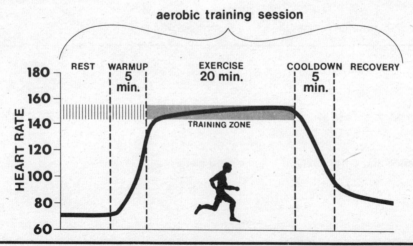

aerobic training session

walk anywhere, let alone run, to get from one place to the next. And in America today, coronary heart disease is the number one killer. Coincidence? Hardly. Lack of exercise, vigorous exercise, is directly related to the rise of heart disease. Running and jogging are not a panacea for heart disease but they can reduce your risks of having a heart attack by strengthening the heart muscle, lowering your body weight, reducing the amount of fat in the blood, and possibly reducing stress and strain.

Before you begin a running or jogging program, you must know what condition your heart and circulatory system is in. The first order of business should be a visit to your physician. With his OK, take the Step Test in Chapter 1 to give you a rough indication of your cardiovascular condition. Another self-testing method is Dr. Kenneth Cooper's 12-minute run/walk test. You simply

Running is the most instinctive form of cardiovascular-pulmonary endurance exercise known.

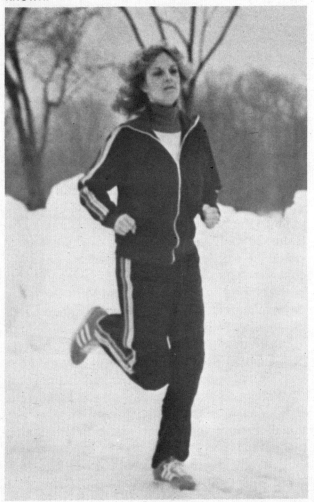

see how much distance you can cover by running and walking in a 12-minute period. If you cover less than a mile, you are in very poor condition. If you traverse 1¾ miles and up in the 12-minute period, you are in excellent condition.

If you are overweight, have diabetes, lower back pain, liver or kidney problems but still want to run, see your doctor before trying the Step Test or Cooper Walk/Run Test. Very likely your doctor can prescribe a walking and/or running program which will best fit your needs.

You may also want to know what the difference is between running and jogging. Not much really. When you run, you move at a pace of roughly 7.5 mph. Jogging is a slightly slower pace—5 mph. If you are a beginner or if your physical fitness rating is poor, you should begin by jogging—after all, the purpose of cardiovascular exercise is rhythmic and sustained activity. If you began by running, you probably could not sustain that fast pace for very long.

With your doctor's OK and an evaluation of your physical fitness condition, you are ready to begin a running or jogging program.

Before You Jog or Run—The Warm-up

The warm-up, which should last about 5 minutes, gradually prepares the body for the exercise to come. Begin with easy stretching exercises and then, as body temperature, circulation, and respiration adjust to the increased activity, move to more vigorous calisthenics (see Chapter 2 for suggested warm-up exercises). Pay particular attention during the warm-up to:

- Stretching the lower back to reduce back problems.
- Stretching hamstring and calf muscles to prevent soreness and reduce the risk of injury.
- Increasing tempo of exercise gradually to adjust body to higher levels of intensity.

Where to Jog or Run

If possible, avoid hard surfaces such as concrete and asphalt for the first few weeks. Running tracks (located at most high schools), grass playing fields, parks and golf courses are recommended. In inclement weather, jog in church, school or YMCA gymnasiums; in protected areas around shopping centers; or in your garage or basement. Varying locations and routes will add interest to your program.

When to Jog or Run

Run whenever it suits your fancy. Some like to get up early and do several miles before breakfast. Others elect to run during the lunch hour, then eat a sandwich at their desk. Many prefer to wait until after work, when running can help cleanse the mind of the day's problems. A few are night owls who brave the dark in their quest for fitness; they are quick to point out that the run and shower help them to sleep like a baby. We would only caution you to avoid vigorous activity 1 or 2 hours after a meal, when the digestive organs require an adequate blood supply, and when any fat in the circulation hastens the risk of clotting.

What to Wear

The most important piece of running "equipment" is the running shoe. Because it is so important, we're covering running shoes separately. Here, we'll talk about the type of clothing you should wear when jogging or running.

Jogging doesn't require fancy clothing. One of running's attractions is the fact that you don't

A jogging suit becomes necessary for winter running/jogging. It's effective to temperatures down to 20 degrees Fahrenheit. (Photo courtesy of Adidas.)

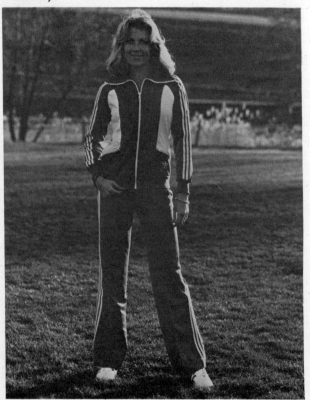

need to spend much money. Nylon or cotton gym shorts and a T-shirt are adequate in summer. For winter running, a sweat suit or jogging suit serves until temperatures fall below 20 degrees Fahrenheit. Some runners prefer cotton thermal knit long underwear under their running shorts. Several layers of lighter apparel are preferable to a single heavy garment. Add gloves and a knit cap in colder temperatures. When the wind blows, a thin nylon windbreaker helps to reduce heat loss. A cap is particularly important in cold weather, since a great deal of body heat is lost through the head.

When temperatures fall below 20 degrees Fahrenheit, you may choose to wear both the underwear and the sweat suit. Many continue to run despite subzero temperatures. There is no danger in doing so provided you are properly clothed, warmed-up, and sensitive to signs of wind chill and frostbite.

Never wear a rubberized sweat suit in any weather. The water lost through perspiration doesn't contribute to long term weight loss, and your body's most effective mode of heat loss is blocked.

Special Clothing for Women

An American Medical Association study of female athletes and the need for special bras showed that every step a runner took caused the breasts to rise and then fall against the chest. Such a movement, the study concluded, always caused soreness. Women athletes have commented that on the occasions when the bouncing isn't pronounced enough to be painful, it's always psychologically uncomfortable.

Since the best custom fit bras for running cost from $20 to $25, some women are reluctant to spend the money. But a well-fitted bra should be considered a necessary part of the woman's running equipment. Since right and left breasts are never identical, a custom fit bra for the serious runner should be considered.

In addition to being individually fitted, the best bras shouldn't have underwires or anything that puts weight on the shoulders. It should limit both up and down and lateral motion and be made of firm, elastic material that's nonabrasive and nonallergenic, with either velcro fastening or a placket to protect the skin from metal fasteners.

There are less expensive substitutes. For those who aren't allergic to synthetics, there's a Warner's bra of firm elastic with adjustable

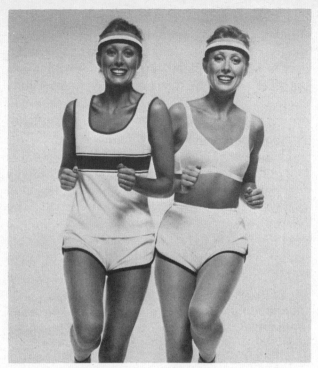

The Running Bra by Formfit Rogers is designed to minimize bounce, skin irritation and collagen tissue breakdown which results in sagging.

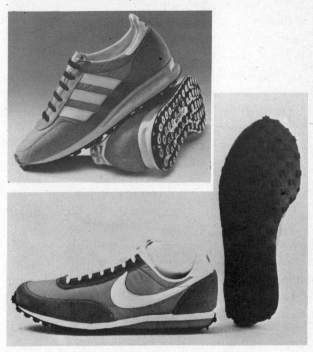

Adidas' Formula I training flat (inset) has a high heel lift which helps relieve strain on the Achilles tendon. Nike's Elite racing flat (below) is designed for the serious competitive runner.

straps. Formfit Rogers recently introduced "The Running Bra" specifically designed for the runner/jogger. Sears, Roebuck & Co. sells their Step-In Sports Bra with an all-around stretch nylon bottom band that holds the bra in place—no fastener is needed.

Running Shoes

Everyone agrees that the most important piece of equipment for a runner is the right pair of shoes. There are many good, durable, well-made running shoes on the market. Probably your best bet for finding the right pair for you is a sporting goods store or shoe store, unless you trade at an exceptional department store. However, few stores carry *all* the well-accepted brands of running shoes. The beginning runner can expect to do a considerable amount of shopping around, particularly in a nonmetropolitan area, in order to find the brand or type of shoe that fits best.

Some runners buy their shoes by mail-order and find their purchases most satisfactory. You don't just send your shoe size and width but also a pencil outline of each foot, since the right and left feet are seldom identical. If the shoes aren't right for you when they arrive, send them back immediately.

If you're trying on running shoes in a store, wear your running socks. If you wear both an inner and outer pair of socks when running, as some runners do, wear both when you're getting fitted. Again, it's a good idea to take with you a pencil outline of each foot. Comparing the bottom of a shoe with your tracing can often show you a great deal about conformity to your foot.

When you try a shoe on, pay special attention to the toe area. Cramped toes can cause trouble. When standing, there should be at least ¾-inch between the tips of your toes and the end of the shoe.

One "must" is foot comfort, so you should walk around the store to ascertain how comfortable—or uncomfortable the shoe is.

Everyone agrees that good foot support is vitally important since your feet will be hitting the ground hard many times during the running session. Nearly all running shoes have some support, but the amount is by no means standard. While it's possible to *add* support after you've bought shoes, it's certainly preferable to have what you want already in the shoe as it comes from the manufacturer.

Training flats, the shoes worn from day to day in running sessions, are considerably heavier than racing flats, which are built light to give a racer greater speed. The racing flats aren't recommended for the less experienced or non-competitive runner.

But even in the training flats, there can be a vast difference in weight. Extra weight can exhaust you on a long run. The lightest weight training flats that fill the bill in other respects will be your best choice.

All-over fit is one of the requirements—and nobody except the wearer can be absolutely sure that a shoe fits him perfectly for running and jogging. A shoe that doesn't come in a variety of widths as well as lengths is one to be wary of.

A shoe must have flexibility, especially in the sole. If the sole doesn't bend easily, the shoe can create great problems for you. Soles should provide both protection and cushioning, while staying flexible. Some shoes have more than one sole—a tough outer sole to fight impact and wear, and one, two, or even three softer inside layers to cushion the foot and absorb the pounding.

Treads on shoe soles vary. Currently, the most popular is the waffle tread, consisting of a series of raised grippers. The waffle tread provides good traction. The grippers absorb the first part of the impact and can consequently be considered part of the cushioning process.

Spikes are recommended only for experienced competitive racers and are definitely much more jarring than rubber treads.

While you might think that a narrow heel would be preferable, it's now been established that wider heels give more stability. The heel should, however, hold the heel of your foot snugly, to avoid blisters. A somewhat elevated heel is now considered preferable. The back of the heel should hit the back of your foot at a comfortable level. If it is too low, the shoe will not provide the support you need. If too high, you will be plagued by blisters.

The upper of the shoe is often the selling feature, simply by eye-appeal, but the upper must be functionally correct, too. It must be firm enough to hold the foot in position but soft enough to be comfortable. Thick seams in an upper can be uncomfortable and irritating.

Uppers come in nylon, leather or a combination of the two. Most runners prefer nylon because of its light weight and the fact that it permits air to circulate more freely. It's also more water-resistant than leather and easier to clean.

Running/Jogging Technique

An upright posture while running conserves energy. Run with your back comfortably straight, your head up, and shoulders relaxed. Bend your arms with hands held in a comfortable position; keep arm swing to a minimum during jogging and slow running. Pumping action increases with speed. Legs swing freely from the hips with no attempt to overstride. Many successful distance runners employ a relatively short stride.

No aspect of running technique is violated more often by neophytes than the footstrike.

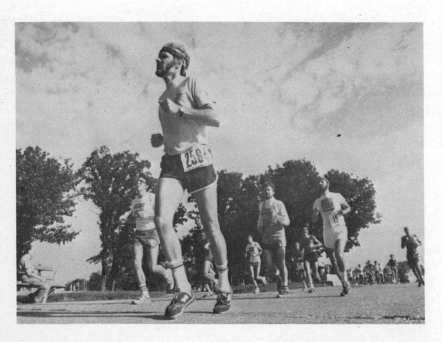

Left—A marathon is probably the most guelling and brutally demanding event a runner can enter. It consists of a 26-mile, 385-yard run, non-stop. Opposite page—During vigorous exercise in a hot, humid environment, sweat rates can approach 3 quarts an hour for short periods. (Photos courtesy Chicago's Mayor Daley Marathon.)

Many newcomers say they can't or don't like to jog. Observation of their footstrike often reveals the reason: they run on the ball of the foot. While appropriate for sprints and short distances, this footstrike is inappropriate for distance runs and will probably result in soreness. The *heel-to-toe* footstrike is recommended for most runners. Upon landing on the heel, the foot rocks forward to push off on the ball of the foot. This technique is the least tiring of all, and a large percentage of successful distance runners use it. The flat-footed technique is a compromise where the runner lands on the entire foot and rocks onto the ball for push-off. Check your shoes after several weeks of running; if you're using the correct footstrike, the outer border of the heel will be wearing down.

Hot Weather Running

At moderate temperatures the body heat generated by exercise or work is easily dissipated. As temperatures increase, the temperature-regulating mechanisms increase perspiration rate to keep the body temperature from climbing above tolerable limits (about 102.5 degrees Fahrenheit). (As perspiration evaporates it cools the body.) When humidity is high, it doesn't evaporate, and no heat is lost. At that point, excessive sweating only contributes to the problem. Perspiration comes from the blood and reduces blood volume. Also, salt and potassium needed by the cells are lost in perspiration.

During work in the heat, it's common to lose more than a quart of sweat an hour. During vigorous exercise in a hot, humid environment, sweat rates can approach 3 quarts an hour for short periods. A good estimate of fluid loss is the body weight difference after work in the heat. Athletes often lose 6-8 pounds in a single workout. Adequate replacement of water, salt and potassium is vital to maintain exercise or work capacity and to avoid heat cramps, heat exhaustion or heat stroke.

To replace salt loss, drink lightly salted water (¼-teaspoon of salt per quart of water), and use the saltshaker at mealtime. Avoid salt tablets. Potassium must be replaced with citrus fruits or juices. Some commercially available drinks supply fluid and electrolyte (inorganic chemicals for cellular reactions) needs. Another approach is to lightly salt lemonade or to drink tomato juice and water (or tomato juice, then water) in volumes comparable to the fluid loss.

The body adjusts or acclimates to work in the heat. Gradual exposure to exercise in a hot environment leads to changes in blood flow, reduced salt loss, and increased perspiration. After 5 to 7 days your heart rate for the same amount of exercise may decline from 180 to 150 beats per minute. Physically fit individuals acclimate more readily to work in the heat, their well-trained circulatory systems make them better suited to its demands. Acclimated individuals should be able to replace salt loss with the saltshaker at meals.

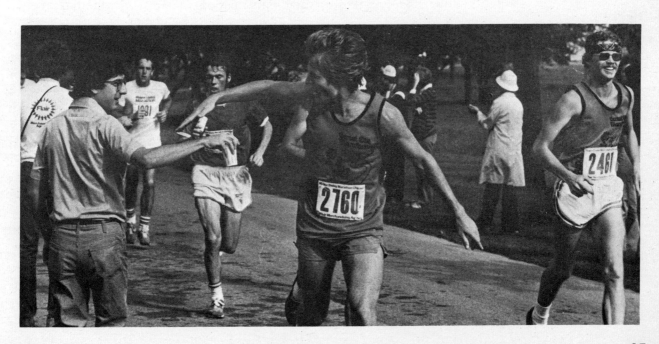

Altitude and Running

As you ascend to higher elevations to run or jog, be aware of limitations imposed on work capacity by reduced oxygen supply.

During the first few weeks of exposure to altitude, your ability to perform is impaired. It can be improved over a period of several weeks by training at that altitude. Altitude acclimatization leads to improved lung function, increased red blood cells and hemoglobin, and increased numbers of capillaries in the working muscles. These changes reduce but never eliminate the effect of altitude on aerobic capacity.

Air Pollution and Running

Avoid exercise in a polluted atmosphere. Carbon monoxide takes the place of oxygen in the red blood cells, which reduces aerobic capacity. Air pollution can:

Irritate airways (bronchitis).

Break down air sacs in lungs (emphysema).

Reduce oxygen transport.

Cause cancer.

One source of pollution can do all these things—the cigarette. It's probably the worst single source of air pollution.

The U.S. Surgeon General has stated that the effects of smoking also may be harmful to the nonsmoker who is exposed to the smoke of cigarettes, cigars, and pipes. Pipe and cigar smoke is particularly unhealthy because it hasn't been inhaled into the smoker's lungs, which helps to filter out some of the harmful ingredients in the smoke.

Running and Jogging Problems

Previously inactive adults often encounter problems when they begin exercising. You'll avoid such problems if you vow to make haste slowly. It may have taken you 10 years to get in the shape you're in and you won't be able to change it overnight. Plan now to make gradual progress. At the start, too little may be better than too much. After several weeks, when your body has begun to adjust to the demands of vigorous effort, you'll be able to increase your exercise intensity.

Another way to avoid exercise problems is to warm-up before each and every exercise session. Careful attention to pre-existing stretching and warming eliminates many of the nagging complications that plague less patient individuals. Never forget to cool down after each workout. In short, prevention is the most effective way to deal with exercise problems.

Blisters: Blisters can be prevented by wearing good, properly fitted shoes. At the first hint of discomfort, cover the area with some moleskin or a large bandage. If you do get a blister, puncture the edge with a sterilized needle to drain the accumulated fluid, treat with an antiseptic, cover with gauze, circle with foam rubber, and go back to work. It's wise to keep the items needed for blister prevention at hand.

Muscle soreness: Soreness, usually due to exercise after long inactivity, may be caused by microscopic tears in the muscle or connective tissue, or to contractions of muscle fibers. It's almost impossible to avoid soreness when you first begin exercising. Minimize it by exercising modestly, at least at first, and by doing mild stretching exercises when soreness does occur. Stretching can be used to relieve soreness and to warm-up for exercise on the following day. Massage and warm muscle temperatures also seem to minimize the discomfort of soreness.

Side stitch: Commonly experienced by the beginner or unconditioned runner. A sharp pain felt just beneath the rib cage, it is thought to be a muscle cramp in the abdominal area, perhaps the diaphragm muscle. If you can stand the pain, keep on running; there is nothing to worry about and it will eventually go away.

Muscle cramps: Cramps are powerful involuntary muscle contractions. Immediate relief comes when the cramped muscle is stretched and massaged. However, that does not remove the underlying cause of the contraction. Salt and potassium are both involved in the chemistry of contraction and relaxation. Cold muscles seem to cramp more readily. It's always wise to warm-up before vigorous effort and to replace salt and potassium lost through sweating in hot weather.

Bone bruises: Hikers and joggers sometimes get painful bruises on the bottoms of the feet. Such bruises can be avoided by careful foot placement and by quality footwear. Cushioned inner soles also help. A bad bruise can linger, delaying your exercise many weeks. There's no instant cure once a bruise has developed, so prevention seems the best advice. Ice may help to lessen discomfort and hasten healing. Padding

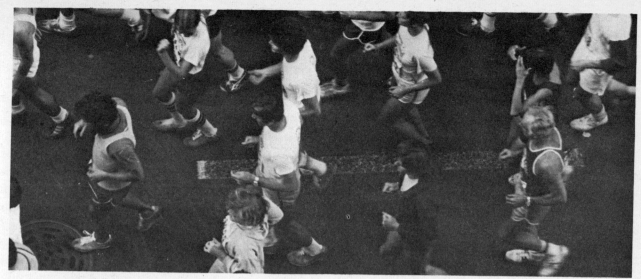

Careful attention to proper warm-up before each jogging/running session will help avoid physical problems. (Photo courtesy of Chicago's Mayor Daley Marathon.)

may allow exercise in spite of the bruise.

Ankle problems: A sprained ankle should be iced immediately. A bucket of ice water in the first few minutes may allow you to work the next day. A serious sprain should be examined by a physician. High-topped gym shoes reduce the risk of ankle sprains in games such as basketball, tennis, handball; low-cuts with thick soles invite sprains. Ankle wraps and tape allow exercise after a sprain, but again, prevention is a more prudent course.

Achilles tendon: Achilles tendon injuries have become quite common. Some high-backed running shoes have been implicated in the rash of *bursa* injuries among runners. The bursa is located beneath the tendon and serves to lubricate its movements. When rubbed long enough, it becomes inflamed. Once inflamed, it may take weeks or months to return to normal. Ice helps, but continued activity is often impossible for several weeks. Rupture of the achilles tendon seems to be more frequent in recent years. Partial rupture occurs when some of the fibers of the tendon are torn. Complete rupture results when the tendon, which connects the calf muscles to the heel, is completely detached. Prevention is the only approach to these problems since surgery is the only cure. An inflammation of the tendon could lead to partial or complete rupture if left untreated or abused. Also, individuals with high serum uric acid levels seem prone to achilles tendon injuries. Those with high levels should have ample warm-up before exercising and should avoid sudden starts, stops, and changes of direction during their exercise.

Shin splints: Pains on the lower portion of the shin bone are known as shin splints. They're caused by a lowered arch, irritated membranes, tearing of muscle from bone, a muscle spasm due to swelling of that muscle, a hairline fracture of the bones of the lower leg, muscle strength imbalance, or other factors. Rest is the best cure for shin splints, although taping or a sponge heel pad seem to help in some cases. Preventive measures include exercises to strengthen shin muscles, gradual adjustment to the rigors of exercise, running on softer surfaces, occasionally reversing direction when running on a curved track, and using the heel-to-toe footstrike.

Knee problems: A knee injury suffered early in life can affect the ability to exercise. For example, a knee injured playing high school football may lead to signs of arthritis in the late 20s or early 30s. Such degenerative changes often restrict the ability to run, ski or engage in other vigorous activities. Those of you with knee problems should consult your physician for ways to relieve the limitations they impose. Some have found that aspirin effectively suppresses the inflammation and pain often associated with exercise. Ice helps to reduce the inflammation and speed your return to activity. Knee problems also can result from improper footstrike, worn shoes, or improper foot support. Repair worn shoes, and if knee problems persist, see a doctor or podiatrist.

Low back pain: Lack of physical activity, poor posture, inadequate flexibility, and weak abdominal or back muscles cause the low back pains that beset millions of Americans. Specific exercises can strengthen one muscle group or stretch another to remove the muscular imbalance and improve the posture. By improving abdominal strength and stretching back muscles the forward tilt of the pelvis can be reduced.

Stressful exercises: Anything that is "perceived" as a threat is stressful. One of the body's responses to stressful situations is the secretion of several "stress" hormones. Associated with this response is an acceleration of the clotting time of the blood. Exercise may be stressful when it's unfamiliar, exhaustive, or highly competitive. Older individuals should begin participating in unfamiliar activities gradually, avoid exhaustion, and postpone competition until fitness and familiarity provide the proper background.

Sudden vigorous exercise: Any sudden vigorous exercise, such as shoveling snow, is a special kind of stress. Failure to warm-up properly leads to cardiac abnormalities caused by an inadequate oxygen supply to the heart. A 5-minute warm-up eliminates the problem.

BICYCLING

Bicycling can be an excellent fitness activity to build cardiovascular endurance. Unlike jogging or running, it is a safe exercise for the obese, overweight or unfit and, like running or jogging, can provide the strenuous type of workout needed to condition the cardiovascular system. You noticed we used the word "can." If you wish to use bicycling as your cardiovascular endurance exercise you *must* cycle over 8 miles per hour for any benefit to take place. How fast you pedal depends on your physical condition and how much work it takes to get your heart beating at your training rate. If you pedal at 10 mph and at the end of 5 minutes haven't reached your training rate, you'll have to pedal faster. Trial and error and pulse checks will tell you when you are working hard enough to effect beneficial results. Like calisthenics, the only resistance you are working against is the weight of your body. To increase that resistance, ride up hills or put your cycle in a gear that offers more resistance.

One other *must* if you have chosen bicycling—flexibility exercises for the hamstring and leg muscles. This can't be over-emphasized. When you pedal, you don't get the maximum extension of the ankle and foot, which can result in a shortened hamstring and a loss of leg flexibility. So prior to cycling and after cycling, flexibility exercises for the hamstring and lower leg should be done. See Chapter 2 for exercises specific to these areas.

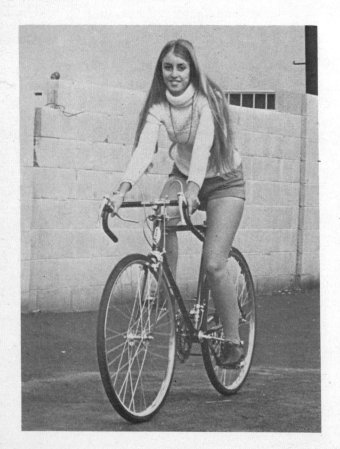

Left and Below—Bicycling can be an excellent cardiovascular endurance exercise. However, you must cycle over 8 miles per hour for any benefit to take place. Like calisthenics, the only resistance you are working against is the weight of your body.

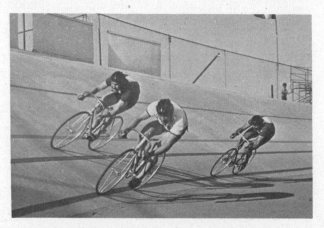

SWIMMING

Swimming is recognized as America's most popular active sport. It is one of the best physical activities for people of all ages and for many persons who are handicapped. Vigorous water activities can make a major contribution to the *flexibility, strength,* and *circulatory endurance* of individuals. With the body submerged in water, blood circulation automatically increases to some extent; pressure of water on the body also helps promote deeper ventilation of the lungs; and with well-planned activity, both circulation and ventilation increase still more.

In order to improve cardiovascular endurance via swimming, you must use one of the five recommended strokes—the crawl, the breaststroke, backstroke, butterfly or side stroke. The swimming strokes should be performed rhythmically and continuously with the swimmer covering about 30 yards a minute. You must swim at your training heart rate for a minimum of 15 minutes for any fitness improvement to take place.

Since each of these swimming strokes utilizes all the major muscles in the body, warm-up exercises for flexibility and strength are extremely important. They will help you avoid being stricken with muscle cramps and soreness during and after your swimming session. You can either pick exercises from Chapters 2 and 3 for flexibility and strength or you can pick from the pool activities which follow. However, whether you choose activities from previous chapters or from those exercises which follow, you should concentrate on back stretching and strengthening exercises. Most swimming strokes cause the back to be in a hyper-extended position. Thus static stretching exercises for the back are highly recommended. One excellent deckside back stretching exercise is to stand with legs apart, extending the hands high over head and reaching as far as possible, holding that position for 5-10 seconds. Then bend the trunk forward and down, flexing the knees, trying to touch the floor. Hold that position for 20-30 seconds and repeat several times.

Aquatic Flexibility Exercises

Increased flexibility work is performed more easily in water because of the lessening of gravitational pull. A person immersed to the neck in water experiences an apparent loss of 90 per-cent of his weight. This means that the feet and legs of a woman weighing 130 lbs. immersed in water only have to support a weight of 13 lbs. Thus, individuals and especially older people with painful joints or weak leg muscles will usually find it possible and comfortable to move in the water. It is much easier to do leg straddle or stride stretches in water than on the floor. Too, many individuals could do leg "bobbing" or jogging in the water who could never do so on land.

Through proper warm-up the body's deep muscle temperature will be raised and the ligaments and connecting tissues stretched, thereby preparing the body for vigorous work. This will help avoid injury and discomfort.

ALTERNATE TOE TOUCH (hamstring muscles)
Standing, in waist-to-chest deep water, swimmer:
1. Raises left leg, bringing right hand toward left foot, looking back and left hand extended rearward.
2. Recover to starting position.
   Repeat.
   Reverse.

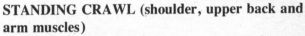

STANDING CRAWL (shoulder, upper back and arm muscles)
Standing in waist-to-chest deep water swimmer:
1. Simulates the overhand crawl stroke by:
   a. Reaching out with the left hand, getting a grip on the water, pressing downward and pulling, bringing the left hand through to the thigh.
   b. Reaching out with the right hand, etc.
   Repeat.

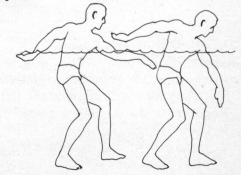

TOE RAISES (lower leg muscles)

Standing in chest-deep water, swimmer:
1. Raises on toes.
2. Lowers to starting position.
   Repeat.
   Accelerate.

WALKING TWISTS (lower back, trunk and leg muscles)

With fingers laced behind neck, swimmer:
1. Walks forward bringing up alternate legs, twisting body to touch knee with opposite elbow.
   Repeat.

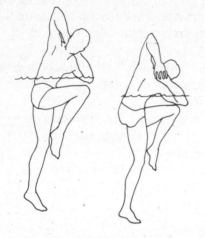

FLAT BACK (lower back muscles)

Standing at side of pool in waist-to-chest deep water, swimmer:
1. Presses back against wall, holding for six counts.
2. Relaxes to starting position.
   Repeat.

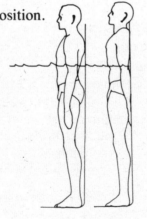

SIDE BENDER (trunk muscles)

Standing in waist-deep water, with left arm at side and right arm over head, swimmer:
1. Stretches, slowly bending to the left.
2. Recovers to the starting position.
   Repeat.
   Reverse to right arm at side and left arm overhead.

STRETCH AND TOUCH (upper back and arm muscles)

Standing, facing wall with arms extended and fingertips approximately 12" from wall, swimmer:
1. With shoulders under water, twists left and tries to touch wall with both hands.
2. Twists right and tries to touch wall with both hands.
   Repeat.

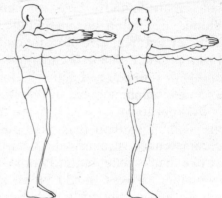

LEG SWING OUTWARD (inner thigh)

Standing with back against poolside, and hands sideward holding gutter, swimmer:
1. Raises left foot as high as possible with leg straight.
2. Swings foot and leg to left side.
3. Recovers to starting position by pulling left leg vigorously to right.
   Repeat.
   Reverses to right leg.
   Repeat.

LEG OUT (leg muscles)

Standing at side of pool with back against wall, swimmer:
1. Raises left knee to chest.
2. Extends left leg straight out.
3. Stretches leg.
4. Drops leg to starting position.
   Repeat.
   Reverse to right leg.

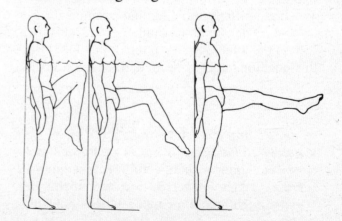

TWIST HIPS (trunk muscles)

Standing, holding on to pool gutter with hands, with back to wall, swimmer:

1. Twists hips to left as far as possible, keeping the upper trunk facing forward.
2. Recovers.
3. Twists hips to right.
4. Recovers.

Aquatic Strength Exercises

TOE BOUNCE (lower leg muscles)

Standing in waist-to-chest deep water with hands on hips, swimmer:

1. Jumps high with feet together through a bouncing movement of the feet.
   Repeat.

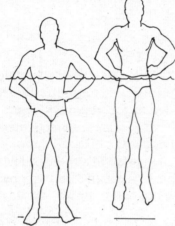

JOGGING IN PLACE (upper and lower leg muscles)

Standing with arms bent in running position, swimmer:

1. Jogs in place.

LEGS TOGETHER ON BACK (inner thigh muscles)

Supine, holding on to pool gutter with hands, legs together and extended with feet about 6" under the water, swimmer:

1. Spreads legs apart as far as possible.
2. Pulls feet and legs vigorously together.
   Repeat.

FRONT FLUTTER KICKING (leg muscles and back muscles)

Lying in a prone position and holding on to side of pool with hand(s), swimmer:

1. Kicks flutter style in which toes are pointed back, ankles are flexible, knee joint is loose but straight and the whole leg acts as a whip.

HIGH BOBBING (leg, arm and shoulder muscles)

In water approximately 1 to 3 feet over the swimmer's head, swimmer:

1. Takes a vertical position, hands extended outward from the sides with palms turned downward. Legs are drawn in position for frog kick.
2. Simultaneously pulls hands sharply to thighs with legs executing frog kick.
3. Inhales at peak of height.
4. Drops with thrust of arms downward with palms turned upward until feet reach bottom of the pool and tucks to a squat position. Exhales throughout this action.
5. Jumps upward with power leg thrust at the same time pulling arms in a breast stroke position downward, causing the head and shoulders to rise high out of water. Exhales during 4 and 5.
6. Inhales and repeats cycles 4 and 5, etc.

POWER BOBBING (leg, arm and shoulder muscles)

Power bobbing is similar to "high bobbing" except that at the top of the upward thrust the hands scull vigorously as the legs flutter and kick. In "power bobbing" the swimmer will

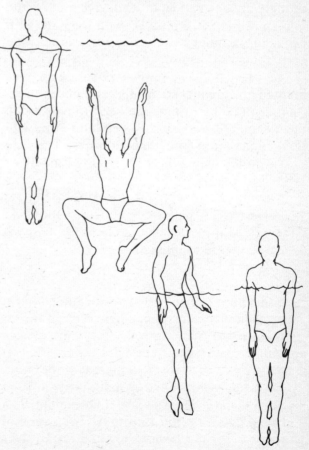

literally blast out of the water exposing all of the body to the hips. Bobbing is a well-rounded workout involving leg power, arm and shoulder work, heavy forced breathing, and rhythmical vigorous action.

Aquatic Cardiovascular-Pulmonary Exercises

Crawl Stroke: The crawl stroke is the fastest of the swimming strokes. For the correct body position in crawl swimming, the body should be a streamlined whole with the body face down in the water and the legs extended and slightly below the surface. The arms move alternately so that as one ends its pull stroke, the other begins its pull stroke. The hand enters the water with the arm extended, elbow slightly bent and held high in the air. When the arm is pulling through the water, the shoulder should be over the elbow and the elbow over the wrist and hand. This position affords the greatest pulling power. As the palm hits the water, you press downward and backward with shoulder and arm muscles for the first third of the stroke, push downward in the middle third and backward during final stroke. Do not push upward after final third—the arm should only be at about a 180-degree arc. As the arm comes out of the water, with the other arm beginning its pulling stroke, the elbow is bent and carried high in the air.

The legs are held fairly straight, with toes pointed and are kicked in a flutter motion. Breathing is done by turning the head to either side during the recovery of the overwater arm, with quick inhalation and then returning the face downward exhaling through the nose, mouth or both.

In performing the crawl, there should be no lateral movement or extreme arching of the back. This will cause imbalance, a decrease in speed and an increase in fatigue.

Breast Stroke: The breast stroke and butterfly are very similar in form but differ primarily in arm action. In the breast stroke, the arms always remain beneath the surface of the water. The two hands are extended together in front of the body, palms facing outward and are pulled outward and backward until the arms are a little more than perpendicular to the body. At the point of maximum spread, the arms are brought together under the chest and extended again quickly.

The kick that accompanies the breast stroke can be of two types—the wedge (frog) kick or the whip kick. The whip kick is generally considered the more efficient of the two. Both are characterized by a "squeezing" action of the legs. The difference is that in the wedge the feet are drawn up to the body, knees bent, and are vigorously kicked outward to the fully extended position. The legs are then drawn together in a "squeezing" fashion. The whip kick is a much narrower kick with the knees kept much closer together and with the legs never reaching the fully extended position.

Breathing is accomplished by raising the head out of the water as the arms are completing their stroke and before they are being brought together underneath the chest.

Butterfly: The butterfly is a competitive swimming stroke and is very strenuous and difficult to master. In the butterfly the arms are above water in the recovery stage, and in the propulsive stage are pressed downward and backward under the body all the way to the hips. They are then lifted in a rotary fashion out of the water, brought forward of body, in fully extended position with palms down, to begin the next stroke.

The kick used with the butterfly can be either the wedge kick or the dolphin or fishtail kick. The dolphin kick, however, must be used if swimming competitively. In the dolphin kick, the legs are kept together and simultaneously move up-and-down in a vertical plane.

Breathing during the butterfly takes place at the end of each stroke with the head raised out of the water for a quick breath and then lowered as the arms are brought forward for the next stroke.

Side Stroke: The side stroke is best known for its use in lifesaving situations and for many people is the preferred stroke for open water swimming because the face remains constantly above water. The body always remains on the side with the arms propelling the body alternately. The under arm begins from a fully extended position and pulls downward below the body to the waist, then bends upward and pushes forward to fully extended position. The upper arm pulls outside the body line, pulling from the chest to the thigh and is brought back to chest level close to the water surface but not above the surface.

The kick used with the side stroke is the scissors kick. The legs open slowly by bending the knees, the underleg moving backward, the upper leg forward, and then are whipped together in a closing movement. The closing action is timed with the finish of the upper arm stroke.

Back Stroke: As in the side stroke, the face in performing the back stroke is always out of the water. In performing the back stroke, keeping the body as streamlined as possible, with legs together and feet pointed is important. There should be a slight bend at the waist in order to get the maximum propulsion from the kicking action of the legs. But if the bend is too pronounced, it will create drag and will make the stroke less effective. Each arm alternately stretches above the head and enters the water directly above and in line with the shoulder with the palms facing outward. When the palm enters the water it is pulled to the thigh. In the first third of the pull, the arm is fully extended, the middle third is done with arm slightly bent and final third with arm in full extension.

The kick used with the back stroke is like that of the crawl stroke. Legs extended, toes pointed, legs moving in up-and-down flutter motion but with the emphasis on the up beat of the kick.

The Slow Progressive Build-Up

Swimming is unique in that age is no hindrance and individuals of varying exercise tolerance levels can utilize this activity to develop organic vigor and to improve flexibility, strength and the blood circulation.

Contrary to an old myth, swimming is compatible with training for other sports. It does not detract from the strength gained through other conditioning activities in the training regimen.

Obviously, individuals in poor condition must work slowly and progressively. It has taken many years for most adults to get out of shape. One should be patient and realize that rebuilding the heart, lungs and body may take a long period of time. A commitment to regularity and gradual build-up will pay off. There may be speed limits but no age limits for either sex. Daily workouts are recommended, but gains can be made with 30-40 minutes of water work 3-5 times per week. Train, don't strain!

ROPE JUMPING

This is such a good exercise that it can be a full-time aerobic fitness activity. The equipment is inexpensive and easy to transport. You can skip rope anywhere, even in a hotel room. The exercise allows a wide range of exercise intensities, and research studies have equated 10 minutes of vigorous rope skipping in cardiovascular benefit to 20 to 30 minutes of jogging.

Rope length is important. It should reach the armpits when held beneath the feet. Commercial skip ropes with ball bearings in the handles are easier and smoother to use, but a length of #10 sash cord from your local hardware store serves quite well.

Rope skipping requires a degree of coordination, and if done inappropriately can quickly raise the heart rate above your training zone. If this happens, walk or jog in place slowly, then resume skipping.

Besides the aerobic benefits, rope skipping can improve your tennis or handball, where rapid footwork is important.

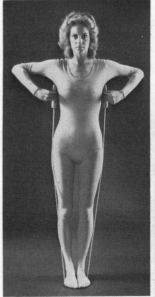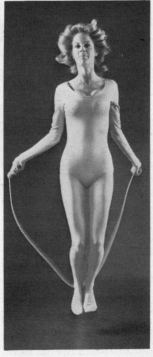

Above and right—Rope jumping can be used as a full-time aerobic exercise. Rope length is important. It should reach the armpits when held beneath the feet.

CHAPTER 5

Total Fitness Programs

IN A TECHNICAL SENSE, total physical fitness can be viewed as a measure of the body's strength, stamina (endurance), and flexibility. In more meaningful personal terms it is a reflection of your ability to work with vigor and pleasure, without undue fatigue, with energy left for enjoying hobbies and recreational activities, and for meeting unforeseen emergencies. It relates to how you look and how you feel—and, because the body is not a compartment separate from the mind, it relates to how you feel mentally as well as physically.

Physical fitness is many-faceted. Basic to it are proper nutrition, adequate rest and relaxation, good health practices, and good medical and dental care.

But these are not enough. An essential element is physical acitivity—exercise for a body that needs it. The following are *total* fitness programs, providing you with complete progressive exercise programs for each level of fitness— poor, average and excellent.

After you reach the level of fitness you have deemed suitable (hopefully Level 5), you can keep yourself fit by continuing the workouts presented in that level. While it is possible to maintain fitness with three workouts a week, you should ideally make exercise a daily habit.

ADULT PHYSICAL FITNESS PROGRAMS

About the Programs—They assume that you have not been engaging recently in consistent, vigorous, all-round physical activity—even though, in daily routines, you have put some muscles to extensive use. Your Personal Physical Fitness Evaluation Chart scores (see Chapter 1) will tell you what your present state of physical fitness is. Unless you are in excellent condition, you should begin with the orientation exercises and progress through all the exercise levels.

The Physical Fitness Programs for men and women are basically the same with but two exceptions: the knee pushup for women is replaced by the standard pushup for men and the number of exercise repetitions and distances for circulatory activities is greater for men.

What the Exercises Are for

There are four general types—**warm-up exercies, conditioning exercises, circulatory activities,** and **cool-down exercises.**

The **warm-up exercises** stretch and limber up the muscles and speed up the action of the heart and lungs, thus preparing the body for greater exertion and reducing the possibility of unnecessary strain.

The **conditioning exercises** are systematically planned to tone-up abdominal, back, leg, arm and other major muscles.

The **circulatory activities** produce contraction of large muscle groups for relatively longer periods than the conditioning exercises—to stimulate and strengthen the circulatory and respiratory systems.

The **cool-down exercises** help gradually to bring your cardiovascular system back down to its normal functioning rate and also help stretch muscles to reduce soreness. The same cool-off exercises outlined here in the Orientation Program will be used after each exercise session and throughoutout the five levels.

When it comes to the circulatory activities, you choose one each workout. Alternately running and walking . . . skipping rope . . . running in place. All are effective. You can choose running and walking on a pleasant day, one of the others for use indoors when the weather is inclement. You can switch about for variety.

How You Progress

A sound physical conditioning program should take into account your individual tolerance — your ability to execute a series of activities without undue discomfort or fatigue. It should provide for developing your tolerance by increasing the work load so you gradually become able to achieve more and more with less and less fatigue and with increasingly rapid recovery.

As you move from level to level, some exercises will be modified so they call for increased effort.

Others will remain the same but you will build more strength and stamina by increasing the number of repetitions.

You will be increasing your fitness another way as well.

At the Orientation Level your objective is to complete all the exercises without a breathing spell in between. If you cannot complete the exercises without taking a breathing spell, stay with the Orientation Program until you can. Then move to Level 1. Also, the first six exercises of the Orientation Program will be used as warm-up exercises throughout the graded levels (Levels 1 thru 5).

At Level 1, your objective will be gradually to reduce, from workout to workout, the "breathing spells" between exercises until you can do the seven conditioning exercises without resting. You will proceed in the same fashion with the more difficult exercises and increased repetitions at succeeding levels.

You will find the program designed—the progression carefully planned—to make this feasible. You will be able to proceed at your own pace, competing with yourself rather than with anyone else—and this is of great importance for sound conditioning. Note: Gradually speeding up, from workout to workout, the rate at which you do each exercise will provide greater stimulation for the circulatory and respiratory systems and also help to keep your workouts short. However, the seven conditioning exercises should not be a race against time. Perform each exercise correctly to insure maximum benefit.

Choosing Your Goal

There is no need to pick the level to which you want to go—now.

Many individuals will be able to advance through the first three levels. While the fourth is challenging, some will be able to achieve it. The fifth is one which only extremely vigorous, well-conditioned persons will reach.

The level of fitness you can reach depends upon your age, your body's built-in potential capacity and previous conditioning. It also depends upon your state of mind; as you know, when you want to do something and believe you can, it is much easier to do than otherwise.

While there will be no dramatic overnight changes, gradually over the next weeks and months, as you progress through the first levels, you will begin to notice a new spring in your step, a new ease with which you accomplish your ordinary daily activities. You will find yourself with more energy left at the end of the working day and a new zest for recreation in the evening. Quite likely, you will be sleeping more soundly than you have slept for many years and waking more refreshed in the morning.

After completing the early levels, you may come to realize that you can—and want to—go further. Go as far as you can.

The important point is that, no matter what level you choose as your goal, you will greatly improve your physical fitness and you will be able to maintain the improvement and continue to enjoy the benefits.

When and How Often to Workout

To be most beneficial, exercise should become part of your daily routine—as much so as bathing, dressing.

Five workouts a week are called for throughout the program.

You can choose any time that's convenient. Preferably, it should be the same time every day—but it doesn't matter whether it's upon arising, at some point during the morning or afternoon, or in the evening.

How Long at Each Level

Your objective at each level will be to reach the point where you can do all the exercises called for, for the number of times indicated, without resting between exercises.

But, start slowly.

It cannot be emphasized enough that by moving forward solidly you will avoid sudden strains and excesses that could make you ache and hold you back for several days.

If you find yourself at first unable to complete any exercises—to do continuously all the repetitions called for—stop when you encounter difficulty. Rest briefly, then take up where you left off and complete the count. If you have difficulty at first, there will be less and less with succeeding workouts.

Stay at each level for at least 3 weeks. If you have not passed the prove-out test at the end of that time, continue at the same level until you do. The prove-out test calls for performing—in three consecutive workouts—the seven conditioning exercises without resting and satisfactorily fulfilling the requirement for one circulatory activity.

A Measure of Your Progress

You will, of course, be able to observe the increase in your strength and stamina from week to week in many ways—including the increasing facility with which you do the exercises at a given level.

In addition, by taking the 4-minute Step Test (Chapter 1, page 6) you can measure and keep a running record of the improvement in your cardiovascular-pulmonary efficiency, one of the most important aspects of fitness.

The immediate response of the cardiovascular system to exercise differs markedly between well-conditioned individuals and others. The test measures the response in terms of pulse rate taken shortly after a series of steps up and down onto a bench or chair. Although it does not take long, it is necessarily vigorous. Stop if you become overly fatigued while taking it.

Your Progress Records

Charts are provided for the Orientation Program and for each of the five fitness levels.

They list the exercises to be done and the goal for each exercise in terms of number of repetitions, distance, etc.

They also provide space in which to record your progress—(1) in completing the recommended 15 workouts at each level, (2) in accomplishing the three prove-out workouts before moving on to a succeeding level, and (3) in the results as you take the Step Test each time.

You do the warm-up exercises and the conditioning exercises along with one circulatory activity for each workout. Following the circulatory activity period, you do the five cooling-off exercises.

Check off each workout as you complete it. The last three numbers are for the prove-out workouts, in which the seven conditioning exercises should be done without resting. Check them off as you accomplish them.

You are now ready to proceed to the next level.

As you take the Step Test—at about 2-week intervals—enter your pulse rate.

When you move on to the next level, transfer the last pulse rate from the preceding level. Enter it in the margin to the left of the new progress record and circle it so it will be convenient for continuing reference.

ORIENTATION PROGRAM

Conditioning Exercises
1. Bend and Stretch

Starting position: Stand erect, feet shoulder-width apart.

Action: Count 1. Bend trunk forward and down, flexing knees. Stretch gently in attempt to touch fingers to toes or floor. Count 2. Return to starting position.

Note: Do slowly, stretch and relax at intervals rather than in rhythm.

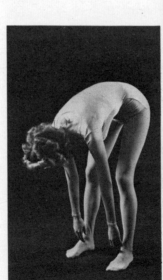
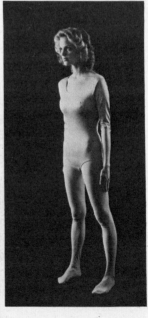

2. Knee Lift

Starting position: Stand erect, feet together, arms at sides.

Action: Count 1. Raise left knee as high as possible, grasping leg with hands and pulling knee against body while keeping back straight. Count 2. Lower to starting position. Counts 3 and 4. Repeat with right knee.

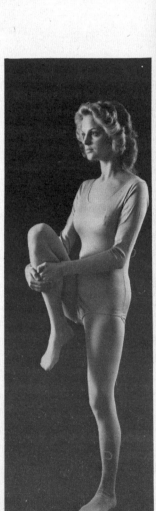
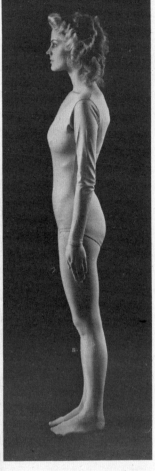

5. Arm Circles

Starting position: Stand erect, arms extended sideward at shoulder height, palms up.

Action: Describe small circles backward with hands. Keep head erect. Do 15 backward circles. Reverse, turn palms down and do 15 small circles forward.

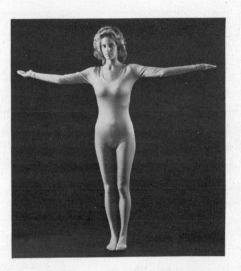

6. Body Bender

Starting position: Stand, feet shoulder-width apart, hands behind neck, fingers interlaced.

Action: Count 1. Bend trunk sideward to left as far as possible, keeping hands behind neck. Count 2. Return to starting position. Counts 3 and 4. Repeat to the right.

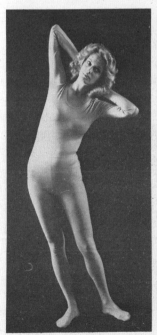
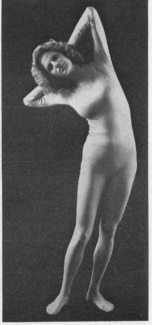

3. Wing Stretcher (see Chapter 2, page 22)

4. Half Knee Bend (see Chapter 2, page 18)

7. Prone Arch (see Chapter 3, page 40)

8. Knee Pushup (Men and Women)

Starting position: Lie on floor, face down, legs together, knees bent with feet raised off floor, hands on floor under shoulders, palms down.

Action: Count 1. Push upper body off floor until arms are fully extended and body is in straight line from head to knees. Count 2. Return to starting position.

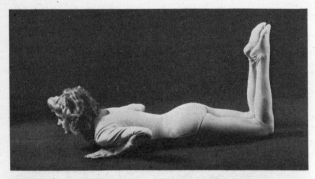

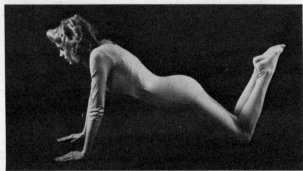

9. Head and Shoulder Curl

Starting position: Lie on back, hands tucked under small of back, palms down.

Action: Count 1. Tighten abdominal muscles, lift head and pull shoulders and elbows off floor. Hold for four seconds. Count 2. Return to starting position.

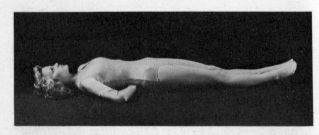

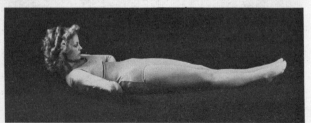

10. Lower Leg Stretch (see Chapter 2, page 17)

Circulatory Activities

Walking: Step off at a lively pace, swing arms and breathe deeply.

Rope: Any form of skipping or jumping is acceptable. Gradually increase the tempo as your skill and condition improve.

Orientation Program Chart

ORIENTATION PROGRAM	GOAL
Conditioning Exercises	*Repetitions*
*1. Bend and Stretch	10
*2. Knee Lift	10 left, 10 right
*3. Wing Stretcher	20
*4. Half Knee Bend	10
*5. Arm Circles	15 each way
*6. Body Bender	10 left, 10 right
7. Prone Arch	10
†8. Knee Pushup	6
9. Head and Shoulder Curl	5
10. Lower Leg Stretch	15

Circulatory Activity (choose 1 each workout)

Walking	½-mile
Rope (skip 15 sec.; rest 60 sec.)	3 series

Cooling-off Exercises (see Chapter 2 for the cooling-off exercises which will be used throughout the graded levels)

1. Neck Circles (page 23)
2. Hamstring Stretch (page 16)
3. Side Twister (page 21)
4. Wing Stretcher (page 22)
5. Side Lunge (page 24)

---

*The first six exercises of the Orientation Program will be used as warm-up exercises throughout the graded levels.

†The Knee Pushup is used by both men and women during the Orientation Program only.

Step Test Record—After completing the Orientation Program, take the 4-minute Step Test (as described in Chapter 1, page 6). Record your pulse rate here:_____. This will be the base rate with which you can make comparisons in the future.

THE FIVE FITNESS LEVELS

LEVEL 1

Conditioning Exercises

1. Toe Touch
Starting position: Stand at attention.
Action: Count 1. Bend trunk forward and down, keeping knees slightly flexed, touching fingers to ankles. Count 2. Bounce and touch fingers to top of feet. Count 3. Bounce and touch fingers to toes. Count 4. Return to starting position.

2. Sprinter
Starting position: Squat, hands on floor, fingers pointed forward, left leg fully extended to rear.
Action: Count 1. Reverse position of feet in bouncing movement, bringing left foot to hands, extending right leg backward—all in one motion. Count 2. Reverse feet again, returning to starting position.

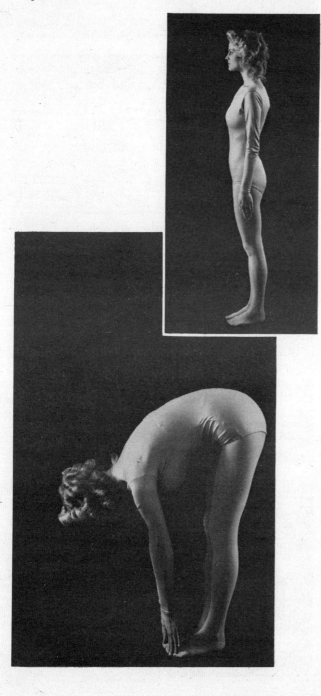

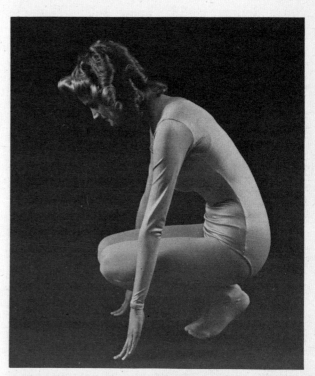

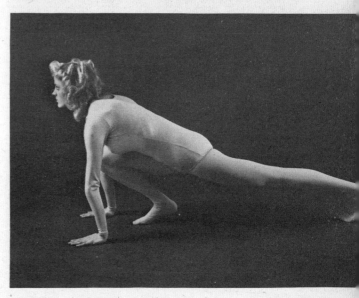

3. Sit and Stretch (see Chapter 2, page 24)

4. Knee Pushup: Women (see Orientation Program)

4. Pushup: Men

Starting position: Lie on floor, face down, legs together, hands on floor under shoulders with fingers pointing straight ahead.

Action: Count 1. Push body off floor by extending arms, so that weight rests on hands and toes. Count 2. Lower the body until chest touches floor.

Note: Body should be kept straight, buttocks should not be raised, abdomen should not sag.

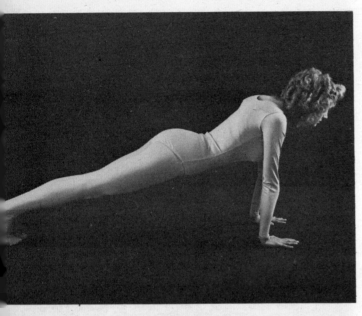

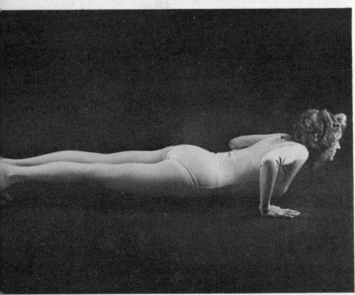

5. Situp (Arms Extended)

Starting position: Lie on back, legs straight and together, arms extended beyond head.

Action: Count 1. Bring arms forward over head, roll up to sitting position, sliding hands along legs, grasping ankles. Count 2. Roll back to starting position.

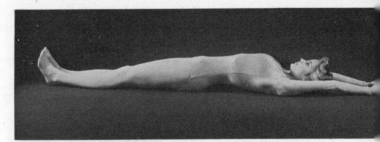

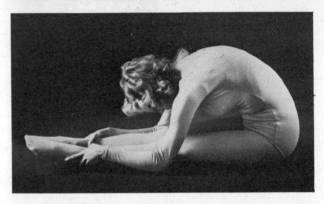

6. Leg Raiser

Starting position: Right side of body on floor, head resting on right arm.

Action: Lift leg about 24″ off floor, then lower it. Do required number of repetitions. Repeat on other side.

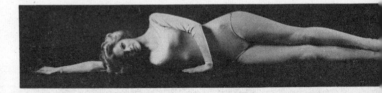

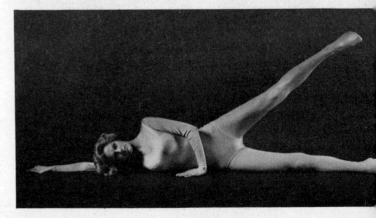

7. Flutter Kick

Starting position: Lie face down, hands tucked under thighs.

Action: Arch the back then flutter kick continuously, moving the legs 8″-10″ apart. Kick from hips with knees slightly bent. Count each kick as one.

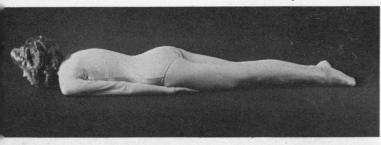

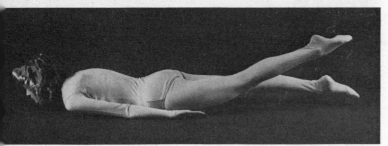

Circulatory Activities

Walking—Maintain a pace of 120 steps per minue for a distance of ½-mile. Swing arms and breath deeply.

Rope—Skip or jump rope using any form. See Level 1 chart for specified times and repetitions.

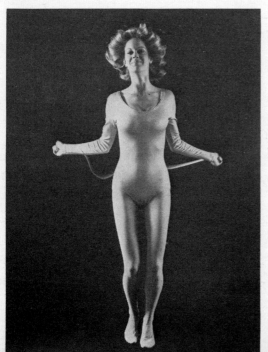

Run in place—Raise each foot at least 4″ off the floor and jog in place. Count 1 each time left foot touches floor. Complete number of running steps called for in chart, then do specified number of straddle hops. Complete 2 cycles of alternate running and hopping for time specified on chart.

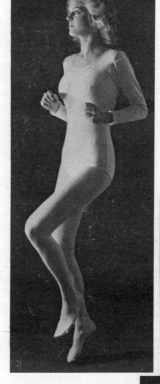

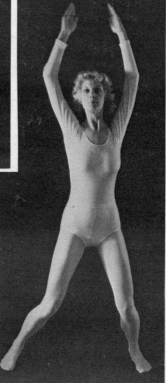

Straddle Hop—

Starting position: At attention.

Action: Count 1. Swing arms sideward and upward, touching hands above head (arms straight) while simultaneously moving feet sideward and apart in a single jumping motion. Count 2. Spring back to starting position. Two counts in one hop.

WOMEN: LEVEL 1   GOAL

Warm-up Exercises   **Exercises 1-6 of Orientation Program**

Conditioning Exercises   **Uninterrupted repetitions**

1. Toe Touch	5
2. Sprinter	8
3. Sit and Stretch	10
4. Knee Pushup	8
5. Situp (Arms Extended)	5
6. Leg Raiser	5 each leg
7. Flutter Kick	20

Circulatory Activity (choose one each workout)

Walking (120 steps a minute)	½ mile
Rope (skip 30 secs.; rest 60 secs.)	2 series
Run in place (run 50; straddle hop 10 — 2 cycles)	2 minutes

Cooling-Off Exercises   **See Orientation Program**

Your progress record	1	2	3	4	5	6	7	8	9	10	11	12	13	14	15
Step Test (pulse)													Prove-out workouts		

MEN: LEVEL 1   GOAL

Warmup Exercises   **Exercises 1-6 of Orientation Program**

Conditioning Exercises   **Uninterrupted repetitions**

1. Toe Touch	10
2. Sprinter	12
3. Sit and Stretch	12
4. Pushup	4
5. Situp (Arms Extended)	5
6. Leg Raiser	12 each leg
7. Flutter Kick	30

Circulatory Activity (choose one each workout)

Walking (120 steps a minute)	1 mile
Rope (skip 30 secs.; rest 60 secs.)	2 series
Run in place (run 60, hop 10 — 2 cycles)	2 minutes

Cooling-Off Exercises   **See Orientation Program**

Your progress record	1	2	3	4	5	6	7	8	9	10	11	12	13	14	15
Step Test (pulse)													Prove-out workouts		

LEVEL 2

Conditioning Exercises

1. **Toe Touch** (see Level 1)

2. **Sprinter** (see Level 1)

3. **Sit and Stretch** (see Chapter 2, page 24)

4. **Knee Pushup: Women** (see Orientation Program)

4. **Pushup: Men** (see Level 1)

5. **Situp (Fingers Laced)**

Starting position: Lie on back, legs bent and feet spread approximately 1″ apart. Fingers laced behind neck.

Action: Count 1. Curl up to sitting position and turn trunk to left. Touch right elbow to left knee. Count 2. Return to starting position. Count 3. Curl up to sitting position and turn trunk to right. Touch left elbow to right knee. Count 4. Return to starting position. Score one situp each time you return to starting position.

6. **Leg Raiser** (see Level 1)

7. **Flutter Kick** (see Level 1)

Circulatory Activities

Jog-Walk—Jog and walk alternately for number of paces indicated on chart for distance specified.

Rope—Skip or jump rope continuously using any form. See Level 2 chart for specified times and repetitions.

Run in place—Raise each foot at least 4″ off floor and jog in place. Count 1 each time left foot touches floor. Complete number of running steps called for in chart, then do specified number of straddle hops. Complete 2 cycles of alternate running and hopping for time specified on chart.

Straddle hop—

Starting position: At attention.

Action: Count 1. Swing arms sideward and upward, touching hands above head (arms straight) while simultaneously moving feet sideward and apart in a single jumping motion. Count 2. Spring back to starting position. Two counts in one hop.

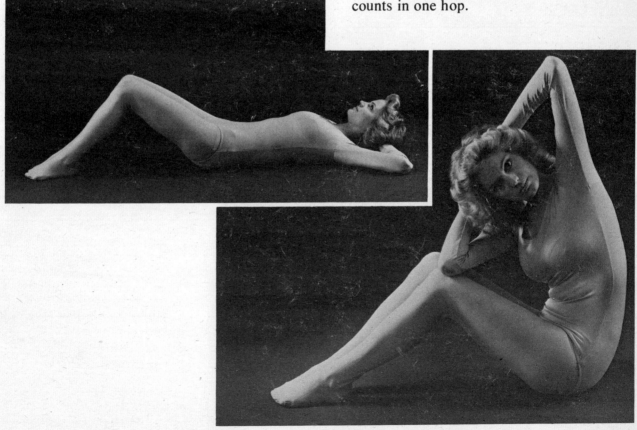

WOMEN: LEVEL 2 | GOAL

Warmup Exercises — Exercises 1-6 of Orientation Program

Conditioning Exercises	Uninterrupted repetitions
1. Toe Touch	10
2. Sprinter	12
3. Sit and Stretch	15
4. Knee Pushup	12
5. Situp (Fingers Laced)	10
6. Leg Raiser	10 each leg
7. Flutter Kick	30

Circulatory Activity (choose one each workout)

Jog-walk (jog 50, walk 50)	½ mile
Rope (skip 30 secs.; rest 60 secs.)	3 series
Run in place (run 80, hop 15 — 2 cycles)	3 minutes

Cooling-Off Exercises — See Orientation Program

Your progress record	1	2	3	4	5	6	7	8	9	10	11	12	13 14 15
Step Test (pulse)													Prove-out workouts

MEN: LEVEL 2 | GOAL

Warm-up Exercises — Exercises 1-6 of Orientation Program

Conditioning Exercises	Uninterrupted repetitions
1. Toe Touch	20
2. Sprinter	16
3. Sit and Stretch	18
4. Pushup	10
5. Situp (Fingers Laced)	20
6. Leg Raiser	16 each leg
7. Flutter Kick	40

Circulatory Activity (choose one each workout)

Jog-walk (jog 100, walk 100)	1 mile
Rope (skip 1min.; rest 1 min.)	3 series
Run in place (run 95, hop 15 — 2 cycles)	3 minutes

Cooling-Off Exercises — See Orientation Program

Your progress record	1	2	3	4	5	6	7	8	9	10	11	12	13 14 15
Step Test (pulse)													Prove-out workouts

LEVEL 3

Conditioning Exercises
1. Toe Touch (see Level 1)

2. Sprinter (see Level 1)

3. Sit and Stretch (see Chapter 2, page 24)

4. Knee Pushup: Women (see Orientation Program)

4. Pushup: Men (see Level 1)

5. Situp (Arms Extended, Knees Up)
Starting position: Lie on back, legs straight, arms extended over head.
Action: Count 1. Sit up, reaching forward with arms encircling knees while pulling them tightly to chest. Count 2. Return to starting position. Do this exercise rhythmically, without breaks in movement.

6. Leg Raiser (see Level 1)

7. Flutter Kick (see Level 1)

Circulatory Activities
Jog-Walk—Jog and walk alternately for number of paces indicated on chart for distance specified.

Rope— Skip or jump rope continuously using any form. See Level 3 chart for specified time and repetitions.

Run in place—Raise each foot at least 4″ off floor and jog in place. Count 1 each time left foot touches floor. Complete number of running steps called for in chart, then do specified number of straddle hops. Complete 2 cycles of alternate running and hopping for time specified on chart.

Straddle Hop—
Starting position: At attention.
Action: Count 1. Swing arms sideward, touching hands above head (arms straight) while simultaneously moving feet sideward and apart in a single jumping motion. Count 2. Spring back to starting position. Two counts in one hop.

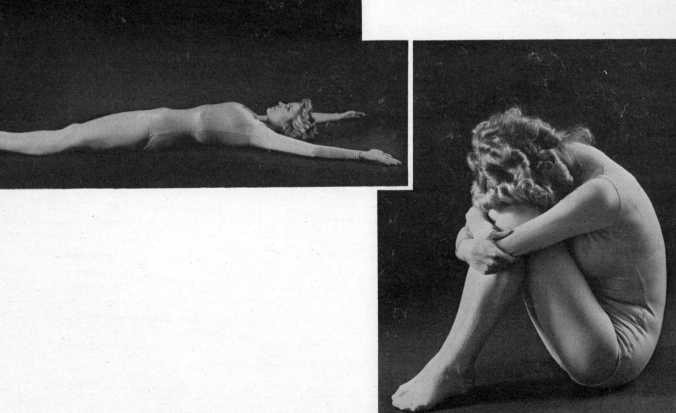

WOMEN: LEVEL 3

GOAL

Warm-up Exercises

Exercises 1-6 of Orientation Program

Conditioning Exercises

Uninterrupted repetitions

1. Toe Touch 20
2. Sprinter 16
3. Sit and Stretch 15
4. Knee Pushup 20
5. Situp (Arms Extended, Knees Up) 15
6. Leg Raiser . . . . 16 each leg
7. Flutter Kick 40

Circulatory Activity (choose one each workout)

Jog-walk (jog 50, walk 50) . . . . ¾ mile
Rope (skip 45 secs.; rest 30 sec.) . . . . 3 series
Run in place (run 110, hop 20 — 2 cycles) . . . . 4 minutes

Cooling-Off Exercises

See Orientation Program

Your progress record	1	2	3	4	5	6	7	8	9	10	11	12	13	14	15
Step Test (pulse)													Prove-out workouts		

MEN: LEVEL 3

GOAL

Warm-up Exercises

Exercises 1-6 of Orientation Program

Conditioning Exercises

Uninterrupted repetitions

1. Toe Touch 30
2. Sprinter 20
3. Sit and Stretch 18
4. Pushup 20
5. Situp (Arms extended, Knees up) 30
6. Leg Raiser . . . . 20 each leg
7. Flutter Kick 50

Circulatory Activity (choose one each workout)

Jog-walk (jog 200; walk 100) . . . . 1½ miles
Rope (skip 1 min.; rest 1 min.) . . . . 5 series
Run in place (run 135, hop 20 — 2 cycles) . . . . 4 minutes

Cooling-Off Exercises

See Orientation Program

Your progress record	1	2	3	4	5	6	7	8	9	10	11	12	13	14	15
Step Test (pulse)													Prove-out workouts		

LEVEL 4

Conditioning Exercises

1. Toe Touch (Twist and Bend)
Starting position: Stand, feet shoulder-width apart, arms extended overhead fingers touching.

Action: Count 1. Twist trunk to right and touch floor inside right foot with fingers of both hands. Count 2. Touch floor outside toes of right foot. Count 3. Touch floor outside heel of right foot. Count 4. Return to starting position, sweeping trunk and arms upward in a wide arc. On the next four counts, repeat action to left side.

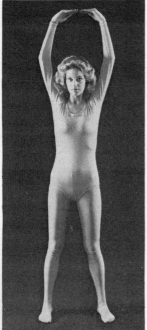

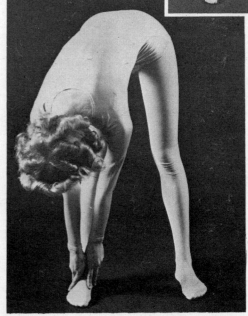

2. Sprinter (see Level 1)

3. Sit and Stretch (Alternate)
Starting position: Sit, legs spread apart, fingers laced behind neck, elbows back.

Action: Count 1. Bend forward to left, touching forehead to left knee. Count 2. Return to starting position. Counts 3 and 4. Repeat to right. Score one repetition each time you return to starting position. Knees may be bent if necessary.

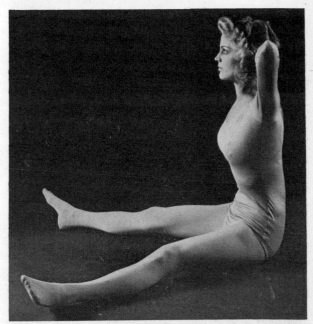

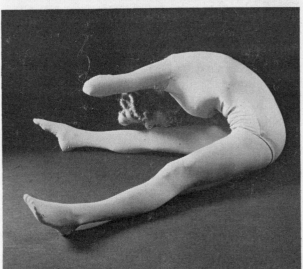

4. Pushup: Women (see Pushup: Men, Level 1)

4. Pushup: Men (see Level 1)

5. Situp (Arms Crossed, Knees Bent)

Starting position: Lie on back, arms crossed on chest, hands grasping opposite shoulders, knees bent to right angle, feet flat on floor.

Action: Count 1. Curl up to sitting position. Count 2. Return to starting position.

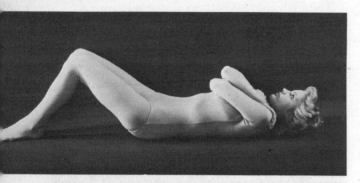

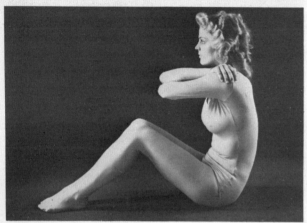

6. Leg Raiser (Whip)

Starting position: Right side of body on floor, right arm supporting head.

Action: Whip left leg up and down rapidly lifting as high as possible off the floor. Count each whip as one. Reverse position and whip right leg up and down.

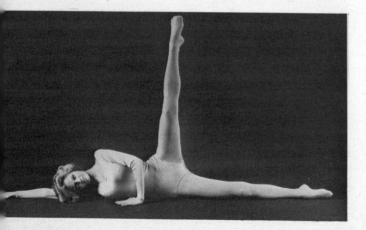

7. Prone Arch (Arms Extended)

Starting position: Lie face down, legs straight and together, arms extended to sides at shoulder level.

Action: Count 1. Arch the back, bringing arms, chest and head up, and raising legs as high as possible. Count 2. Return to starting position.

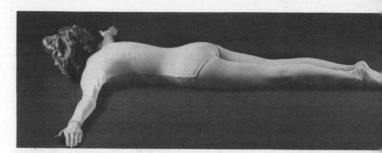

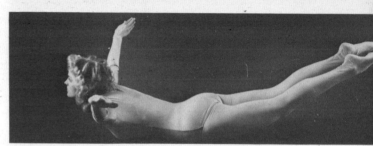

Circulatory Activities

Jog-Walk—Jog and walk alternately for number of paces indicated on chart for distance specified.

Rope—Skip or jump rope continuously using any form. See Level 4 chart for specified times and repetitions.

Run in place—Raise each foot at least 4″ off floor and jog in place. Count 1 each time left foot touches floor. Complete number of running steps called for in chart, then do specified number of straddle hops. Complete 2 cycles of alternate running and hopping for time specified on chart.

Straddle Hop—

Starting position: At attention.

Action: Count 1. Swing arms sideward and upward, touching hands above head (arms straight) while simultaneously moving feet sideward and apart in a single jumping motion. Count 2. Spring back to starting position. Two counts in one hop.

WOMEN: LEVEL 4 GOAL

| **Warm-up Exercises** | **Exercises 1-6 of Orientation Program** |

Conditioning Exercises — **Uninterrupted repetitions**

1. Toe Touch (Twist and Bend) .... 15 each side
2. Sprinter 20
3. Sit and Stretch (Alternate) 20
4. Pushup 8
5. Situp (Arms Crossed, Knees Bent) 20
6. Leg Raiser (Whip) .... 10 each leg
7. Prone Arch (Arms Extended) 15

Circulatory Activity (choose one each workout)
Jog-walk (jog 100; walk 50) .... 1 mile
Rope (skip 60 secs.; rest 30 secs.) .... 3 series
Run in place (run 145, hop 25 — 2 cycles) .... 5 minutes

Cooling-Off Exercises — **See Orientation Program**

Your progress record	1	2	3	4	5	6	7	8	9	10	11	12	13	14	15
Step Test (pulse)													Prove-out workouts		

MEN: LEVEL 4 GOAL

| **Warm-up Exercises** | **Exercises 1-6 of Orientation Program** |

Conditioning Exercises — **Uninterrupted repetitions**

1. Toe Touch (Twist and Bend) .... 20 each side
2. Sprinter 28
3. Sit and Stretch (Alternate) 24
4. Pushup 30
5. Situp (Arms Crossed, Knees Bent) 30
6. Leg Raiser (Whip) .... 20 each leg
7. Prone Arch (Arms Extended) 20

Circulatory Activity (choose one each workout)
Jog .... 1 mile
Rope (skip 90 secs.; rest 30 secs.) .... 3 series
Run in place (run 180; hop 25 — 2 cycles) .... 5 minutes

Cooling-Off Exercises — **See Orientation Program**

Your progress record	1	2	3	4	5	6	7	8	9	10	11	12	13	14	15
Step Test (pulse)													Prove-out workouts		

LEVEL 5

Conditioning Exercises

1. Toe Touch (Twist and Bend) (see Level 4.)

2. Sprinter (See Level 1.)

3. Sit and Stretch (Alternate) (see Level 4.)

4. Pushup: Women (see Pushup: Men, Level 1)

4. Pushup: Men (see Level 1)

5. Situp (Fingers Laced, Knees Bent)
Starting position: Lie on back, fingers laced behind neck, knees bent, feet flat on floor.
Action: Sit up, turn trunk to right, touch left elbow to right knee. Count 2. Return to starting position. Count 3. Sit up, turn trunk to left, touch right elbow to left knee. Count 4. Return to starting position. Score one each time you return to starting position.

6. Leg Raiser (On Extended Arm)
Starting position: Body rigidly supported by extended right arm and foot. Left arm is held behind head.
Action: Count 1. Raise left leg high. Count 2. Return to starting position slowly. Repeat on other side. Do required number of repetitions.

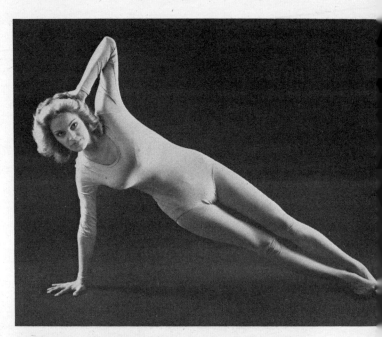

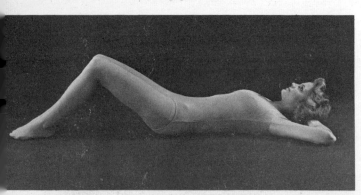

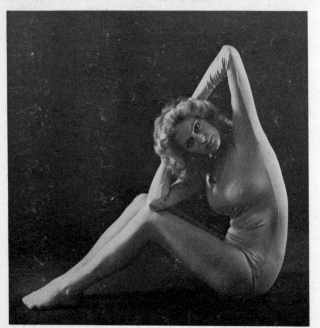

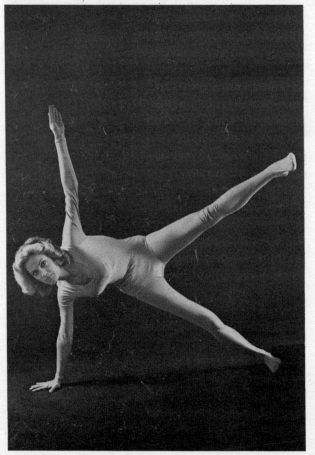

7. Prone Arch (Fingers Laced)

Starting position: Lie face down, fingers laced behind neck.

Action: Count 1. Arch back, legs and chest off floor. Count 2. Extend arms fully forward. Count 3. Return hands to behind neck. Count 4. Flatten body to floor.

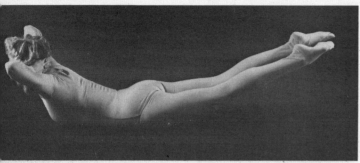

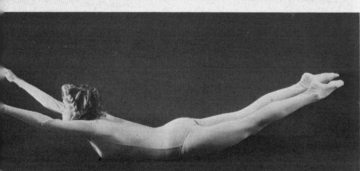

Circulatory Activities

Jog Run—Jog and run alternately for distance specified on chart.

Rope—Skip or jump rope continuously using any form. See Level 5 chart for specified times and repetitions.

Run in place—Raise each foot at least 4″ off floor and jog in place. Count 1 each time left foot touches floor. Complete number of running steps called for in chart, then do specified number of straddle hops. Complete 2 cycles of alternate running and hopping in time specified on the chart.

Straddle Hop—

Starting position: At attention.

Action: Count 1. Swing arms sideward, touching hands above head (arms straight) while simultaneously moving feet sideward and apart in a single jumping motion. Count 2. Spring back to starting position. Two counts in one hop.

ALTERNATIVE WATER ACTIVITIES

The water exercises described below can be used as replacements for the circulatory activities of the basic program. The goals for each of the five levels are shown in the chart below.

Swimming is one of the best physical activities for people of all ages—and for many of the handicapped.

With the body submerged in water, blood circulation automatically increases to some extent, pressure of water on the body also helps promote deeper ventilation of the lungs; and with well-planned activity, both circulation and ventilation increase still more.

WOMEN					
Level	1	2	3	4	5
Bobs	10	15	20	50	100
Swim	5 min	10 min	15 min	—	—
Interval swimming	—	—	—	25 yds (Repeat 10 times)	25 yds (Repeat 20 times)

MEN					
Level	1	2	3	4	5
Bobs	10	15	25	75	125
Swim	5 min	10 min	15 min	—	—
Interval swimming	—	—	—	25 yds (Repeat 20 times)	50 yds (Repeat 20 times)

Bobbing—

Starting position: Face out of water.

Action: Count 1. Take a breath. Count 2. Submerge while exhaling until feet touch bottom. Count 3. Push up from bottom to surface while continuing to exhale. Three counts to one bob.

Swimming—

Use any one of the five strokes described in Chapter 4, pages 72-73. Swim continuously for the time specified.

Interval Swimming—

Use any type of stroke. Swim moderately fast for distance specified (30 yards a minute is recommended). You can then either swim back slowly to starting point or get out of pool and walk back. Repeat specified number of times.

91

WOMEN: LEVEL 5   GOAL

Warm-up Exercises   **Exercises 1-6 of Orientation Program**

Conditioning Exercises   **Uninterrupted repetitions**

1. Toe Touch (Twist and Bend)	25 each side
2. Sprinter	24
3. Sit and Stretch (Alternate)	26
4. Pushup	15
5. Situp (Fingers Laced, Knees Bent)	25
6. Leg Raiser (On Extended Arm)	10 each leg
7. Prone Arch (Fingers Laced)	25

Circulatory Activity (choose one each workout)

Jog-run	1 mile
Rope (skip 2 min.; rest 45 secs.)	2 series
Run in place (run 180, hop 30 — 2 cycles)	6 minutes

Cooling-Off Exercises   **See Orientation Program**

Your progress record	1	2	3	4	5	6	7	8	9	10	11	12	13	14	15
Step Test (pulse)													Prove-out workouts		

MEN: LEVEL 5   GOAL

Warm-up Exercises   **Exercises 1-6 of Orientation Program**

Conditioning Exercises   **Uninterrupted repetitions**

1. Toe Touch (Twist and Bend)	30 each side
2. Sprinter	36
3. Sit and Stretch (Alternate)	30
4. Pushup	50
5. Situp (Fingers Laced, Knees Bent)	40
6. Leg Raiser (On Extended Arm)	20 each leg
7. Prone Arch (Fingers Laced)	30

Circulatory Activity (choose one each workout)

Jog-run	3 miles
Rope (skip 2 min.; rest 30 secs.)	2 series
Run in place (run 216, hop 30 — 2 cycles)	6 minutes

Cooling-Off Exercises   **See Orientation Program**

Your progress record	1	2	3	4	5	6	7	8	9	10	11	12	13	14	15
Step Test (pulse)													Prove-out workouts		

ADULT WALK-JOG-RUN PROGRAMS

Your fitness prescription gives you a great deal of freedom to tailor a personal fitness program to meet your specific fitness, work or recreation goals. You have a wide choice of exercises, and there are many options as far as the length of time you want to exercise and the intensity of that activity. Some of you, particularly those with a new-found interest in fitness, may prefer a more detailed, step-by-step approach. For this reason, some walk-jog-run programs are included.

We'll describe programs for three levels of ability: a **starter program** for those in poor fitness categories, an **intermediate program** for those in the average fitness category, and an **advanced program** for those in the excellent fitness category.

Before you begin any of the walk-jog-run activities, you should do a series of warm-up exercises. Use the warm-up exercises outlined in the Adult Physical Fitness Programs for Men and Women. If, after completing these exercises, your heart beat rate is not at your training level, run in place or jump rope until you achieve your heart beat training level.

After you complete a walk-jog-run session, follow it with a cooling-off period using the exercises outlined in the Adult Physical Fitness Programs. A gradual cool-down after your aerobic exercise is as important as the warm-up. Complete rest immediately after exercise causes blood to pool in the veins and slows the removal of metabolic waste products. Soreness, cramps or more serious cardiovascular complications may follow. Walking or easy jogging continues the pumping action of the muscles, promoting circulation and speeding recovery. A few minutes spent stretching also helps avoid soreness.

Never rush from a vigorous workout into a hot shower! The flow of blood to recently exercised muscles combined with the flow to the skin to dissipate heat may result in inadequate flow to the brain or heart. *Always* cool down after a workout.

STARTER PROGRAMS

Take the *walk test* to determine your exercise level.

Walk Test: The object of this test is to determine how many minutes (up to 10) you can walk at a brisk pace, on a level surface, without undue difficulty or discomfort.

If you can't walk for 5 minutes, begin with Walking Program A.

If you can walk more than 5 minutes, but less than 10, begin with the third week of Walking Program A.

If you can walk for the full 10 minutes, but are somewhat tired and sore as a result, start with Walk-Jog Program B. If you can breeze through the full 10 minutes, you're ready for bigger things. Wait until the next day and take the 10-minute *Walk-Jog Test*.

Walk-Jog Test: In this test you alternately walk 50 steps (left foot strikes ground 25 times) and jog 50 steps for a total of 10 minutes. Walk at the rate of 120 steps a minute (left foot strikes the ground at 1-second intervals). Jog at the rate of 144 steps a minute (left foot strikes ground 18 times every 15 seconds).

If you can't complete the 10-minute test, begin at the third week of Program B. If you can complete the 10-minute test, but are tired and winded as a result, start with the last week of Program B before moving to Program C. If you can perform the 10-minute Walk-Jog Test without difficulty, start with Program C.

Walking Program A

Week	Activity (every other day at first)
1	Walk at a brisk pace for 5 minutes, or for a shorter time if you become uncomfortably tired. Walk slowly or rest for 3 minutes. Again walk briskly for 5 minutes, or until you become uncomfortably tired.
2	Same as Week 1, but increase pace as soon as you can walk 5 minutes without soreness or fatigue.
3	Walk at a brisk pace for 8 minutes, or for a shorter time if you become uncomfortably tired. Walk slowly or rest for 3 minutes. Again walk briskly for 8 minutes, or until you become uncomfortably tired.
4	Same as Week 3, but increase pace as soon as you can walk 8 minutes without soreness or fatigue.

When you've completed Week 4 of Program A, begin at Week 1 of Program B.

Walk-Jog Program B
Week   Activity (four times a week)
1   Walk at a brisk pace for 10 minutes, or for a shorter time if you become uncomfortably tired. Walk slowly or rest for 3 minutes. Again, walk briskly for 10 minutes, or until you become uncomfortably tired.
2   Walk at a brisk pace for 15 minutes, or for shorter time if you become uncomfortably tired. Walk slowly for 3 minutes.
3   Jog 10 seconds (25 yards). Walk 1 minute (100 yards). Do 12 times.
4   Jog 20 seconds (50 yards). Walk 1 minute (100 yards). Do 12 times.

When you've completed Week 4 of Program B, begin at Week 1 of Program C.

Jogging Program C
Week   Activity (five times a week)
1   Jog 40 seconds (100 yards). Walk 1 minute (100 yards). Do 9 times.
2   Jog 1 minute (150 yards). Walk 1 minute (100 yards). Do 8 times.
3   Jog 2 minutes (300 yards). Walk 1 minute (100 yards). Do 6 times.
4   Jog 4 minutes (600 yards). Walk 1 minute (100 yards). Do 4 times.
5   Jog 6 minutes (900 yards). Walk 1 minute (100 yards). Do 3 times.
6   Jog 8 minutes (1,200 yards). Walk 2 minutes (200 yards). Do 2 times.
7   Jog 10 minutes (1,500 yards). Walk 2 minutes (200 yards). Do 2 times.
8   Jog 12 minutes (1,760 yards). Walk 2 minutes (200 yards). Do 2 times.

INTERMEDIATE PROGRAM (JOG-RUN)

If you've followed the starter program or are already reasonably active, you're ready for the Intermediate Program. You're able to jog 1 mile slowly without undue fatigue, rest 2 minutes, and do it again. Your sessions consume about 250 calories.

You're ready to increase both the intensity and the duration of your runs. You'll begin jogging 1 mile in 12 minutes, and when you finish this program you may be able to complete 3 or more miles at a pace approaching 8 minutes a mile. Each week's program includes three phases—the **basic workout, longer runs (overdistance),** and

shorter runs (underdistance). If a week's program seems too easy, move ahead; if it seems too hard, move back a week or two. Remember to make a warm-up and a cooling-off part of every session.

Week 1
Basic Workout (Monday, Thursday)
1 mile in 11 minutes; active recovery (walk). Run twice.
Underdistance (Tuesday, Friday)
¼- to ½-mile slowly.
½-mile in 5 minutes 30 seconds. Run twice (recover between repeats).
¼-mile in 2 minutes 45 seconds. Run 4 times (recover between repeats).
Jog ¼- to ½-mile slowly.
Overdistance (Wednesday, Saturday or Sunday)
2 miles slowly. (Use the Talk Test: Jog at a pace that allows you to converse.)

Week 2
Basic Workout (Monday, Thursday)
1 mile in 10 minutes 30 seconds; active recovery. Run twice.
Underdistance (Tuesday, Friday)
¼- to ½-mile slowly.
½-mile in 5 minutes.
¼-mile in 2 minutes 30 seconds. Run 2 times (recover between repeats).
¼-mile in 2 minutes 45 seconds. Run 2 times (recover between repeats).
220 yards in 1 minute 20 seconds. Run 4 times (recover between repeats).
¼- to ½-mile slowly.
Overdistance (Wednesday, Saturday or Sunday)
2¼ miles slowly.

Week 3
Basic Workout (Monday, Thursday)
1 mile in 10 minutes, active recovery. Run twice.
Underdistance (Tuesday, Friday)
¼- to ½-mile slowly.
½-mile in 4 minutes 45 seconds.
¼-mile in 2 minutes 30 seconds. Run 4 times (recover between repeats).
220 yards in 1 minute 10 seconds. Run 4 times (recover between repeats).
100 yards in 30 seconds. Run 4 times (recover between repeats).
¼- to ½-mile slowly.
Overdistance (Wednesday, Saturday or Sunday)
2½ miles slowly.

Week 4

Basic Workout (Monday, Thursday)

1 mile in 9 minutes 30 seconds; active recovery. Run twice.

Underdistance (Tuesday, Friday)

¼- to ½-mile slowly.

½-mile in 4 minutes 45 seconds. Run twice (recover between repeats).

¼-mile in 2 minutes 20 seconds. Run 4 times (recover between repeats).

220 yards in 1 minute. Run 4 times (recover between repeats).

¼- to ½-mile slowly.

Overdistance (Wednesday, Saturday or Sunday)

2¾ miles slowly.

Week 5

Basic Workout (Monday, Thursday)

1 mile in 9 minutes; active recovery. Run twice.

Underdistance (Tuesday, Friday)

¼- to ½-mile slowly.

½-mile in 4 minutes 30 seconds.

¼-mile in 2 minutes 20 seconds. Run 4 times (recover between repeats).

220 yards in 60 seconds. Run 4 times (recover between repeats).

100 yards in 27 seconds. Run 4 times (recover between repeats).

¼- to ½-mile slowly.

Overdistance (Wednesday, Saturday or Sunday)

3 miles slowly.

Week 6

Basic Workout (Monday, Thursday)

1½ miles in 13 minutes 30 seconds; active recovery. Run twice.

Underdistance (Tuesday, Friday)

¼- to ½-mile slowly.

½-mile in 4 minutes 30 seconds. Run twice (recover between repeats).

¼-mile in 2 minutes 10 seconds. Run 4 times (recover between repeats).

220 yards in 60 seconds. Run 4 times (recover between repeats).

100 yards in 25 seconds. Run twice (recover between repeats).

¼- to ½-mile slowly.

Overdistance (Wednesday, Saturday or Sunday)

3 miles slowly; *increase pace* last ¼-mile.

Week 7

Basic Workout (Monday, Thursday)

1½ miles in 13 minutes; active recovery. Run twice.

Underdistance (Tuesday, Friday)

¼- to ½-mile slowly.

½-mile in 4 minutes 15 seconds. Run twice (recover between repeats).

¼-mile in 2 minutes. Run 4 times (recover between repeats).

220 yards in 55 seconds. Run 4 times (recover between repeats).

¼- to ½-mile slowly.

Overdistance (Wednesday, Saturday or Sunday)

3½ miles slowly; always increase pace near finish.

Week 8

Basic Workout (Monday, Thursday)

1 mile in 8 minutes; active recovery; run 1 mile in 8 minutes 30 seconds; active recovery; repeat (total of 3 miles).

Underdistance (Tuesday, Friday)

¼- to ½-mile slowly.

½-mile in 4 minutes. Run twice (recover between repeats).

¼-mile in 1 minute 50 seconds. Run 4 times (recover between repeats).

220 yards in 55 seconds. Run 4 times (recover between repeats).

100 yards in 23 seconds. Run 4 times (recover between repeats).

¼- to ½-mile slowly.

Overdistance (Wednesday, Saturday or Sunday)

3¾ miles slowly.

Week 9

Basic Workout (Monday, Thursday)

1 mile in 8 minutes. Run 3 times (recover between repeats).

Underdistance (Tuesday, Friday)

¼- to ½-mile slowly.

½-mile in 3 minutes 30 seconds.

¼-mile in 1 minute 45 seconds. Run 4 times (recover between repeats).

220 yards in 50 seconds. Run 4 times (recover between repeats).

100 yards in 20 seconds. Run 4 times (recover between repeats).

50 yards in 10 seconds. Run 4 times (recover between repeats).

¼- to ½-mile slowly.

Overdistance (Wednesday, Saturday or Sunday)
4 miles slowly.

Week 10
Basic Workout (Monday, Thursday)
1½ miles in 12 minutes. Run twice (recover between repeats).
Underdistance (Tuesday, Friday)
¼- to ½-mile slowly.
½ mile in 3 minutes 45 seconds. Run 3 times (recover between repeats).
¼-mile in 1 minute 50 seconds. Run 6 times (recover between repeats).
220 yards in 45 seconds. Run twice (recover between repeats).
¼- to ½-mile slowly.
Overdistance (Wednesday, Saturday or Sunday)
4 miles; increase pace last ½-mile

Week 11
Basic Workout (Monday, Thursday)
1 mile in 7 minutes 30 seconds. Run 3 times (recover between repeats).
Underdistance (Tuesday, Friday)
¼- to ½-mile slowly.
½-mile in 3 minutes 50 seconds. Run 4 times (recover between repeats).
¼-mile in 1 minute 45 seconds. Run 4 times (recover between repeats).
220 yards in 45 seconds. Run 2 times (recover between repeats).
¼- to ½-mile slowly.
Overdistance (Wednesday, Saturday or Sunday)
Over 4 miles slowly (more than 400 calories per workout).

Week 12
Basic Workout
1½ miles in 11 minutes 40 seconds.
You've achieved the fitness level of excellent. Proceed to the advanced aerobic fitness program.

ADVANCED PROGRAM
This section is for the well-trained runner. We'll provide some suggestions for advanced training, but keep in mind there is no single way to train. If you enjoy underdistance training, by all means use it. If you find that you prefer overdistance, you'll like the suggestions offered here.

Long, slow distance running seems to be the ideal way to train. It combines the features of overdistance and underdistance with a minimum of discomfort. Simply pick up the pace as you approach the end of a long run, and you'll receive an optimal training stimulus. Moreover, since the speed work is limited to a short span near the end of the run, discomfort is brief.

Consider the following suggestions:
• Always warm-up before your run.
• Use the Excellent Fitness Heart Rate Training Zone (see page 12).
• Vary the location and distance of the run day by day (long-short; fast-slow; hilly-flat; hard-easy).
• Set distance goals.
    Phase 1: 20 miles a week
    Phase 2: 25 miles a week (ready for 3- to 5-mile road races)
    Phase 3: 30 miles a week
    Phase 4: 35 miles a week (ready for 5- to 7-mile road runs)
    Phase 5: 40 miles a week
    Phase 6: 45 miles a week (ready for 7- to 10-mile road races)
    Phase 7: More than 50 miles a week (consider longer races such as the marathon — 26.2 miles)
• Don't be a slave to your goals, and don't increase weekly mileage unless you enjoy it.
• Run 6 days a week if you enjoy it; otherwise, try an alternate day schedule with longer runs.
• Try one long run (not over one-third of weekly distance) on Saturday or Sunday.
• Try two shorter runs if the long ones seem difficult—5 + 5 instead of 10.
• Keep records if you like — you'll be surprised! Record date, distance, comments. Note resting pulse, body weight. At least annually, check your performance over a measured distance to observe progress (use a local road race or the 1½-mile-run test). Check your fitness score on the Step Test several times a year.
• Don't train with a stopwatch. Wear a wristwatch so you'll know how long you've run.
• Increase speed as you approach the finish of a run.
• Always cool down after a run.